Restoring You

INTESTINAL FLORA

"The ancient healing traditions stated that all diseases could be traced back to improper digestion. And the gut is where one needs to begin. Simply put: proper gut flora brings radiant health; depleted flora causes disease. Why? Because the gut stabilizes the immune system, preventing food allergies and autoimmune diseases; the gut is considered the 'seat of digestion,' where all nutrients are absorbed from the foods you eat; and the gut is also known as the 'brain of the brain,' since the vast majority of the neurotransmitters for the brain are made in the gut. Heal your gut and watch your health return, slowly but surely. Read this book to find out how."

MARIANNE TEITELBAUM, AUTHOR OF
HEALING THE THYROID WITH AYURVEDA

"Much more attention is being paid to the intestinal microbiome as being the culprit behind so many health conditions, from depression to ADHD to poor immunity. In Christopher Vasey's new book *Restoring Your Intestinal Flora,* he sets out an easy-to-follow plan to not only restore this vital organ but also detoxify the wrong kinds of bacteria. This is a must-read book for someone who understands that the gut is the real foundation of health."

ELISA LOTTOR, PH.D., HMD., AUTHOR OF
THE MIRACLE OF REGENERATIVE MEDICINE

"In a society increasingly plagued by inflammatory conditions and digestive disorders, Dr. Vasey's pearls of wisdom on restoring intestinal flora make for a wonderful and interesting read, as well as essential. Referred to as our second brain, the gut is responsible for producing 90 percent of the body's serotonin, a critical neurochemical responsible for inducing positive mental health. This book is a must-read for both mental and physical well-being."

EMMA MARDLIN, PH.D., CONSULTANT, THERAPIST, TRAINER, AND AUTHOR OF *OUT OF YOUR COMFORT ZONE* AND *MIND BODY DIABETES TYPE 1 AND TYPE 2*

"*Restoring Your Intestinal Flora* by Christopher Vasey, N.D, is well written, easily understood, and thoroughly researched on the role of intestinal flora on the digestive system. This book makes several important suggestions to improve your gut health that could have positive impacts on your overall health."

KEDAR N. PRASAD, PH.D., AUTHOR OF *FIGHT DIABETES WITH VITAMINS AND ANTIOXIDANTS* AND *FIGHT ALZHEIMER'S WITH VITAMINS AND ANTIOXIDANTS*

Restoring Your
INTESTINAL FL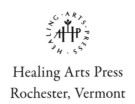RA

The Key to Digestive Wellness

Christopher Vasey, N.D.

Translated by Jon E. Graham

Healing Arts Press
Rochester, Vermont

Healing Arts Press
One Park Street
Rochester, Vermont 05767
www.HealingArtsPress.com

Healing Arts Press is a division of Inner Traditions International

Originally published in French under the title *Je reconstruis ma flore intestinale, c'est parti!*
by Éditions Jouvence, www.editions-jouvence.com, info@editions-jouvence.com
First U.S. edition published in 2021 by Healing Arts Press

Note to the reader: *This book is intended as an informational guide. The remedies,
approaches, and techniques described herein are meant to supplement, and not to be a
substitute for, professional medical care or treatment. They should not be used to treat a serious
ailment without prior consultation with a qualified health care professional.*

Cataloging-in-Publication Data for this title is available from the Library of Congress

ISBN 978-1-64411-093-5 (print)
ISBN 978-1-64411-094-2 (ebook)

Printed and bound in the United States by Versa Press, Inc.

10 9 8 7 6 5 4 3 2 1

Text design and layout by Virginia Scott Bowman
This book was typeset in Garamond Premier Pro with Nexa used as the display typeface

To send correspondence to the author of this book, mail a first-class letter to the author c/o
Inner Traditions • Bear & Company, One Park Street, Rochester, VT 05767, and we will
forward the communication, or contact the author directly at **www.christophervasey.ch.**

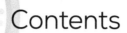

Contents

Introduction

I regularly have problems with my digestion and I suffer from bloating. I often have diarrhea, which alternates with spells of constipation. I was prescribed a treatment with antibiotics, and ever since then I have not been feeling well. I have fungal infections that cause me a lot of inconvenience. I am beginning to develop intolerance to certain foods. I tend to catch colds and flu easily. I often feel a lack of energy. I am always feeling tired and subject to mood swings. Sometimes I even have problems with depression . . .

Stop! All of these disorders, as varied as they are, can be traced back to a single origin: your intestinal flora.

Recent studies have shown that the intestinal flora performs a large number of functions—many more than previously thought. More than our digestion depends on this flora. The intestinal transit, the body's ability to detoxify and fight off infections, our resistance to allergies and inflammation, and even our vitality and joy in life all require beneficial flora. Many diseases can get a foothold once the intestinal flora begins to deteriorate. The problem is that in the modern world the gut is confronted by many threats. These threats are not outside dangers we can't control, but are linked to both our dietary habits (refined foods that are sterilized and low in fiber) and the ways in which we deal with health issues (overuse of antibiotics). These are factors against which we can take effective action, and this book will show you how.

The first part of the book explains what the populations of intestinal flora are and describes all the functions they perform, what things can weaken the flora, and what diseases can arise as a result of that weakening.

The second part of the book is more practical. You will learn how to support the intestinal flora with the ingestion of prebiotics (high-fiber foods that provide the essential nutrients required by the intestinal flora) and how to reinforce the intestinal flora by taking probiotics (foods or supplements that are high in the bacteria that facilitate regeneration of the gut flora).

The means of repairing the intestinal flora that I am presenting here are simple, effective, and easy for anyone to apply.

Self-Diagnosis:
How Healthy Is My Gut?

I eat very few fruits and vegetables.	☐ Yes	☐ No
I don't include yogurt or cheese in my daily diet.	☐ Yes	☐ No
I eat primarily white bread and pasta.	☐ Yes	☐ No
My digestion is slow and difficult.	☐ Yes	☐ No
I often suffer from gas and bloating.	☐ Yes	☐ No
Infections such as colds or cystitis are a recurring theme in my life.	☐ Yes	☐ No
I suffer from yeast or other fungal infections.	☐ Yes	☐ No
I have food allergies.	☐ Yes	☐ No
I have been diagnosed with candida.	☐ Yes	☐ No
Despite all my efforts, I find it difficult to lose weight.	☐ Yes	☐ No
I often feel a lack of energy.	☐ Yes	☐ No
I suffer from mood swings.	☐ Yes	☐ No

Analysis of Results

How many *yes* answers did you have?

0–3: Your intestinal flora is doing well but it would be a good idea to get to know it better in order to keep it healthy.

4–7: Your intestinal flora is experiencing difficulties. This is the time to begin applying the advice provided in this book.

8 or more: It is urgent that you rebuild your intestinal flora and start working on it immediately.

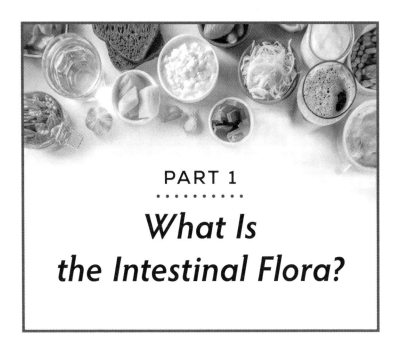

PART 1

· · · · · · · · · · ·

What Is the Intestinal Flora?

■ ■ ■

Our planet Earth is inhabited by a countless number of different kinds of microorganisms. Our whole environment is filled with them. They are in the ground, the air, the water, and even in the ice. For the most part we cannot see them with the naked eye, but they are critical to every aspect of life as we know it. Nowhere is this more true than in the human digestive tract, where intestinal flora help control digestion, prepare food for absorption, break down toxins, prevent the growth of harmful bacteria, and more. The human body literally could not live without the intestinal flora.

There are up to a thousand species of microorganisms in the human gut microbiome, interacting and functioning as a single additional organ. They are essential for our health, but under certain conditions may also be capable of causing disease. It is our responsibility—and in our best interest—to help them stay in balance.

1

Microorganisms and Intestinal Flora

Microorganisms are everywhere; there is not a single place that is spared their presence. In the human body a large number of microorganisms live on our skin and on the mucous membranes of our hollow organs, such as the stomach and intestines. These populations are normal and include all the bacterial flora of our body. They are assigned different names depending on where they are located, so we have buccal (oral cavity) flora, pulmonary flora, vaginal flora, and cutaneous (skin) flora. There are also the bacteria that we are going to focus on in this book: the flora in the intestines.

The word *flora* used in this context may come as a surprise to some readers, as it is generally used to designate the various flowers that grow in a specific region. However, the word is also used to designate all the bacteria inhabiting a given region of the body.

? **Did You Know?**

In everyday speech we use the term *intestinal flora,* but scientists use the word *microbiota,* which includes not only bacteria but also fungi, archaea, and viruses present in the digestive system.

THE FORMATIVE PROCESS
OF THE INTESTINAL FLORA

The intestinal, or gut, flora of human beings plays a major role in the proper functioning of the body. It is an indispensable link in the various stages of the digestive process, as it synthetizes nutrients, neutralizes toxins, and so forth. It is such a fundamental element of our health that the body would be incapable of carrying on without it. However, at the time of birth the newborn human being does not have any. A fetus's digestive tract is sterile, meaning it is entirely flora free. So how does the microbiome come into being? Microorganisms enter the emerging infant from the outside—from the birth canal, the breast, and human touch—to populate the newborn's intestinal tract.

The first microorganisms enter the body through the air inhaled by the newborn through the nose into the respiratory system. When they enter the body they settle in the mucous membranes of the nose, travel from there into the throat, and then further into the body.

Another entranceway is the mouth. The newborn's mouth makes contact with many things besides air that have microorganisms, such as its own fingers, bedding, and the skin of the mother. These microorganisms then migrate into the intestines.

The primary agency for entrance into the body is food, which is loaded with microorganisms. The first food of the newborn human being is mother's milk. A nursing baby ingests not only the milk but the bacteria it contains as well. As mentioned earlier, once inside the body these microbes travel into the intestines. Among these is lactobacillus, the principal bacteria that will populate the intestine.

Like all living things, microorganisms can survive only in an environment that offers favorable conditions for their development. The temperature and amount of moisture must be suitable, and the environment must provide the sustenance they need in sufficient quantities.

Some microorganisms will die once they enter the digestive tract because the conditions are too adverse. Others will simply travel through and be expelled from the body in the stool, because the living conditions they require cannot be met in the digestive tract. But a percentage of the microorganisms that have entered will find their ideal living conditions with an abundant supply of food. They will take up permanent residence, and when they multiply, they will colonize the intestine and form that organ's flora.

? Did You Know?

Mother's milk is ideal for the development of a newborn's intestinal flora. Between 1960 and 1970, when nursing fell out of fashion, many babies were fed infant formula. The resulting deficiencies of their intestinal flora were the cause of a variety of health problems. It was the realization of the true source of these disorders that prompted a return to breast milk and the benefits it confers. Since nursing is not always an option, scientists have tried to apply these benefits to infant formula by adding live bacteria to make it mimic breast milk more closely.

The increase in the number of microorganisms of the early intestinal flora is quite rapid. Forty-eight hours after birth the first stools contain a high level of microorganism content, but not much diversity. After a week the variety of microorganism species is higher, as is the total population. This composition remains stable from this point throughout the entire period the child continues to drink breast milk.

Once the child is weaned and solid food has replaced mother's milk, the composition of the intestinal flora changes. New microorganisms entering the digestive tract expand the number of species already present. A significant number of new foods offer nutrients that sustain them and make it easier for them to multiply. Thereafter their numbers increase greatly.

A VERY LARGE POPULATION

The population of microorganisms in the microbiota is extremely large. It is not counted in thousands of individuals but trillions. The human intestinal flora is composed of one hundred trillion microorganisms (10^{13}). It is about ten times the number of cells in the human body.

If someone wished to gather all the intestinal microorganisms in a single container, this vessel would have to be able to contain one to two quarts. The weight of all these microorganisms would be anywhere from two to seven pounds.

The ecosystem of the microbiota hosts more than four hundred different species of bacteria. But one single species of bacteria can include a large number of subgroups, or serotypes. For example the bacteria *Escherichia coli* (better known as E. coli) can be broken down into more than two hundred different serotypes, some of which produce a toxin but many of which are innocuous.

The microorganisms that populate the intestines are tiny—roughly the size of a micron, which is 0.001 of a millimeter. Comparing them to a single hair gives a better idea of their size. Bacteria and fungi are one thousand times smaller than the thickness of a hair. One cubic millimeter, about the size of a medium salt crystal, can contain one hundred million microorganisms.

☝ Good to Know

- The gut is home to bacteria, yeasts, fungi, archaea, and viruses.
- There are many more bacteria than other micro-organisms.
- Archaebacteria in the gut serve unique digestive functions.
- Most viruses don't cause disease.

MULTIPLICATION
OF MICROORGANISMS

Every day numerous microorganisms are carried away by the stool and thereby removed from the intestinal region. Based on some estimates, the bulk of all these microorganisms together would account for half the weight of the stool. In order to maintain the population of the intestinal flora, the eliminated microorganisms must be replaced constantly with new ones. This is easily achieved for two reasons:

- A great many bacteria are introduced into the body via food every time we eat.
- Bacteria multiply very quickly.

Bacteria have a distinctive method of reproducing that allows their descendants to multiply quickly. A "mother cell" divides into two and thus gives birth to two new cells,

.	1 bacterium
..	2 bacteria
....	4 bacteria
....	8 bacteria
....	16 bacteria
....	32 bacteria
....	64 bacteria
....	
	128 bacteria

Cellular multiplication
(Bacteria are single-celled microorganisms.)

called "daughter cells." During this process the mother cell dies. When they divide in turn, the two daughter cells also die but each gives birth to two new daughter cells. And so it continues. The number of descendants does not increase by one unit per generation, but doubles each time: 2, 4, 8, 16, 32, and so forth. The speed with which bacteria reproduce is thus extremely rapid. It is even faster when one takes into consideration that unlike human beings, for whom a new generation appears every twenty years or so, new generations of bacteria generally appear every fifteen to sixty minutes.

Lactobacillus and *Bifidobacterium,* the bacteria that have the largest presence in the gut, have an average speed of reproduction: a new generation every hour. In twenty hours they produce one million descendants. The multiplication is even quicker for E. coli: a new generation is produced every twenty minutes, or one million individuals every seven hours.

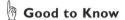 **Good to Know**

The body loses a portion of its intestinal flora on a daily basis, but it is constantly being replaced by new bacteria produced by this same flora.

ARE BACTERIA DANGEROUS?

Bacteria—particularly "germs"—have a reputation of being dangerous. Indeed, they can infect us and make us seriously ill. How is it that the body can offer a home to so many bacteria, and yet they are beneficial?

The answer is that there are billions of different types of bacteria on the planet, but only a minority are pathogenic. All the others have a beneficial role to play. They can be compared to tiny invisible workers whose activity is essential for creating and breaking down matter. The survival of plants and animals hinges entirely on the microbial world.

?　Did You Know?

In nature it is bacteria that give life to the inert minerals in the soil and make it possible for plants to assimilate these minerals (nitrogen, phosphorus, and sulfur). Bacteria are also responsible for the decomposition of dead plants and animals. The tissues of the latter contain a host of substances that can be reused. In order for them to be recycled, they need to be freed from the organic structures holding them. Bacteria break down tissue into smaller particles that are then reabsorbed into the life cycle.

The bacteria of the intestinal flora use the simple substances found in the alimentary bolus to synthesize vitamins, amino acids, and so on. They also break down food particles that have not been sufficiently digested (amino acid chains) or cannot be digested by the digestive juices (plant fiber). Finally, they destroy toxins and poisons by rendering them harmless.

The human body gains a huge advantage from the bacteria of the intestinal flora, and they in turn are beneficiaries of the body. Every day the intestines provide nourishing food residue and a warm, moist environment that is essential for their survival.

☝ Good to Know

A relationship in which two organisms of different species (in this case we are looking at the bacteria that live in the intestines and the human being) both benefit from the presence of the other is called a "symbiotic relationship." The bacteria that contribute to the advantages of this relationship are known as "saprophytes," as opposed to the bacteria that have an adverse effect on human beings, which are called "pathogens."

DISTRIBUTION BY LEVEL

The distribution of bacteria is not uniform throughout the digestive tract. In the mouth the amount is average (about three hundred million per ounce of fluid). In the stomach, on the other hand, it is extremely low (thirty thousand per ounce). The high acidity of the gastric juices kills a number of the bacteria that travel through it, but a certain number do survive and find their way into the intestines. Once there they multiply and their numbers increase sharply. There are three billion per ounce in the first part of the small intestine (the jejunum) and three hundred to three trillion per ounce in the second half of the small intestine (the ileum) and colon.

The distribution of the various types of microorganisms in the intestines occurs naturally based on the characteristics of each type of microorganism.

Among the relatively few microorganisms in the stomach and proximal small intestine we find aerobic bacteria, which need oxygen to survive and thus are found in the duodenum and jejunum, as air from the stomach carries easily into this area. Anaerobic bacteria do not need oxygen to survive and proliferate in the more remote areas that have little oxygen, therefore in the lower half of the small intestine and in the colon.

In order to live and thrive in a segment of the intestine, bacteria do not merely have to travel to the area in question but must be able to take root when they arrive; in other words, attach themselves to the walls of the intestine. As it

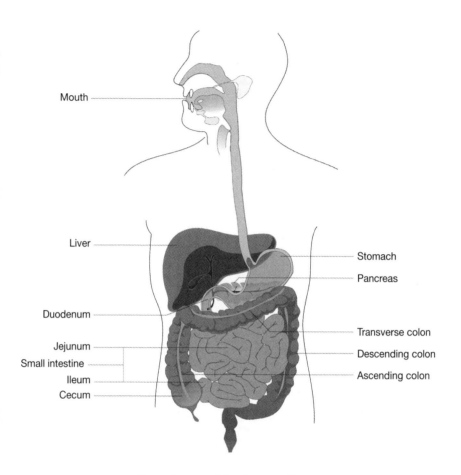

Distribution of the digestive flora

happens, if the intestines have no desire to house certain bacteria, the intestinal mucous membranes release lymphocytes that will attack them and drive them away. Bacteria that are unable to attach to the surface of the walls cannot become part of the intestinal flora or contribute to its maintenance and growth. They are carried out of the body by the stool.

The bacteria that attach themselves to the walls of the intestine stay behind to renew and maintain the microbiota.

In order to find a place in which to settle, bacteria also have to find an available location. The territories that can offer them habitation are the source of intense competition. Countless bacteria cohabitate at every level of the intestine. When there are too many in a particular area or they are entrenched, new bacteria will not be able to find any place in which to settle.

In addition to its normal healthy population of bacteria, the intestinal flora can temporarily offer shelter to pathogenic invaders, but they are not considered part of the intestinal flora.

☝ Good to Know

There are three components of the intestinal flora:

- The dominant population of the flora that are stable and affixed to the intestinal walls (this includes 99 percent of the bacteria)
- The subdominant population of the flora, which are variable and more or less rooted (0.9 percent of the bacteria)
- The fluctuating population of the flora, microorganisms that are simply passing through and do not become attached to the intestinal walls (0.1 percent of the bacteria)

TO EACH HIS
OWN INTESTINAL FLORA

There is no standard composition of microbiota common to all human beings. Every individual has a unique microbiota. There are around fifty bacteria common in 90 percent of the population, but there can be another three hundred and fifty that vary from one individual to the next. The level of yeast and other fungi also varies from one individual to another.

The composition of the microbiota varies not only in the types of microorganisms but also the quantity. Some microbial populations are more numerous than others because they find food in the intestines that is more suitable for their needs.

🎓 What We've Learned

An extremely large number of bacteria, archaea, fungi, viruses, and yeasts reside in our intestines. All together these microorganisms form our microbiota. Far from being a threat to our health, they are necessary for the proper functioning of our bodies.

2

The Functions of Intestinal Microorganisms

Intestinal microorganisms are not unwelcome guests that the body has to tolerate. To the contrary, their activity is beneficial to the body in a variety of ways. Although the contribution of each microorganism is minimal, the combined efforts of billions of them are extremely helpful (and necessary!) to the body.

In addition to supporting the immune system, which is so important that it will be the subject of its own chapter, the microbiota supports the physical organism in many different ways. Here are its primary functions:

DIGESTIVE FUNCTION

Before the cells of the body can benefit from the nutrients we eat, our foods must be broken down into particles that are small enough to cross through the intestinal walls and be transported by the blood to the cells. This preparatory work takes place during digestion.

Digestive juices secreted by the stomach, liver, pancreas, and intestines all help to break down food into particles: proteins into amino acids, fats into fatty acids, starch into glucose, and so on.

Although the digestive juices are capable of performing an immense part of this transformative work, they cannot do it all. Some of the nutrients in a food item can elude them. There are three reasons for this:

- Some foods are made up of more or less hard fiber that contains nutrients but is impervious to the action of the digestive juices.
- Fiber forms the framework of the foods' tissues and can hold nutrients captive.
- When some food particles reach the intestine, they are still too bulky for the digestive enzymes to have any meaningful effect on them. The digestive processes have not been fully completed.

Are the nutrients unaffected by digestion doomed to remain unused? No, the microorganisms of the intestine carry out the transformations that are still necessary. They produce enzymes that break down the fibers and framework of the tissues, and they reduce the volume of the large particles. Nutrients that are still highly useful will be released by this process: amino acids, carbohydrates, vitamins, and so forth.

These final transformations of food are not performed by intestinal bacteria as a favor to their human hosts but for their own benefit. In fact, they also need to feed themselves to survive, and their food is the remnants of the foods we eat. When they attack these remnants, they free the remaining nutrients trapped inside, which allows them to survive. The rest of the nutrients will be absorbed by the body, and in quantities that allow us to benefit from them.

The Two Major Categories of Bacteria

The digestive processes are carried out with the help of two major types of bacteria that live in different regions of the intestines: bacteria of fermentation and bacteria of putrefaction.

Bacteria of Fermentation

The word *ferment* comes from Latin, meaning "to boil, to cause to rise," and originally referred to leavening with yeast. Bacteria of fermentation break down food in the second half of the small intestine—the ascending colon and more than half of the transverse colon, releasing heat (energy) in the process. Maximum concentration is found in the area of the cecum and the ascending colon. The bacteria present in the largest number here are ones we hear a lot about: *Lactobacillus acidophilus* and *Bifidobacterium*.

The fermentation processes of these bacteria target the long carbohydrate chains, such as starch, but also the soft fibers of

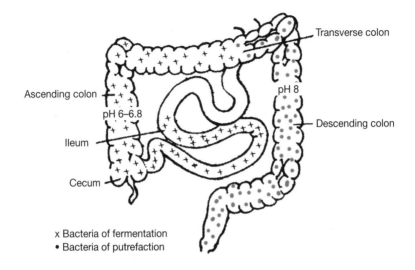

Allocation of the intestinal flora

grains, fruits, vegetables, fruit peels, ribs of leafy plants, stringy parts of leek-like plants, and so on.

? Did You Know?

Lactobacillus bacteria do not get their name because they come from milk, but because their activity produces lactic acid. Sources of lactobacillus include both animal products (milk, yogurt) and some vegetables.

Fibers such as pectin, inulin, and lignin cannot be processed by our digestive juices. However, the bacteria of the microbiota are able to transform them thanks to the fermentation processes they trigger. This fragments the fibers into smaller particles, which frees the nutrients they contain.

✍ Good to Know

While the soft fiber of grains—the lignin—is broken down by intestinal flora, the hard fiber—bran, which is made of cellulose—is not.

The process in the human body is similar to the one that occurs in the digestive tract of herbivores. Cows, for example, ingest an enormous quantity of fiber in their grass consumption, but their digestive juices need an assist from the large intestinal flora of their microbiota.

Termites also consume a great deal of fiber in the wood they ingest, but their digestive juices need help as well. They have very active intestinal flora that break down the hard fibers of the wood.

The leaves that fall from deciduous trees in autumn form a thick carpet on the ground. The bacteria in the soil causes them to decompose and be transformed into humus. The same process happens in a garden compost pile of dead flowers, grass clippings, food scraps, and so on. When these scraps are attacked by the bacteria of fermentation, they are transformed into beautiful, rich soil.

But let's return to the human digestive tract. One consequence of the fermentation that takes place in the process of breaking down foods is the production of acidic substances: lactic, acetic, propionic, butyric, succinic, and carbonic acids. These substances acidify the portion of the intestines where the bacteria of fermentation are traditionally established. They create a slightly acidic environment (pH 6 to 6.8) that encourages the bacteria of fermentation and allows them to thrive.

Bacteria of Putrefaction

The word *putrefaction* also comes from Latin and means "to make rotten, to break down or decompose." This flora occupies a small part of the transverse colon and all of the descending colon, where it is most heavily concentrated.

The bacteria of putrefaction break down any undigested particles of food that come their way. These are not fibers, having already been transformed by fermentation higher up in the intestines, but the residue of proteins (meats, fish, eggs) and starches (bread, pasta, rice).

The decomposition of food particles through putrefaction produces such wastes as ammonia, indole, skatol, phenols, hydrogen sulfide, ptomaine, and so forth. Because they are alkaline, these substances make the descending colon an alkaline environment (pH 8), which is beneficial for the development of the bacteria of putrefaction.

Flora	Area of Habitation	Environmental pH
Flora of fermentation	Small intestine, ascending colon, transverse colon (first half)	Slightly acidic (pH 6 to 6.8)
Flora of putrefaction	Transverse colon (second half), descending colon	Alkaline (pH 8)

The combined action of the bacteria of fermentation and putrefaction allows the complete digestion of food to take place as it works its way through the different segments of the intestines. Although the bacteria are simply completing the work of the digestive juices, they are absolutely essential for the physical organism, which could not function without them.

ABSORPTION OF NUTRIENTS

Once the nutrients provided by food have been made available through the digestive process, they still need to be absorbed so that cells can benefit from them. This absorption takes place in the intestinal mucous membranes, or to be more exact, the tiny, finger-like intestinal villi that carpet the walls of the small intestine.

? Did You Know?

From 90 to 95 percent of the absorption of nutrients takes place in the second half of the small intestine, and only 5 to 10 percent in the terminal part of the colon.

When the small intestine is empty or nearly empty, the intestinal walls fold back over themselves forming rugae, or ridges, that will expand when filled with food. The ridges lessen the possibilities for absorption as there are fewer exposed openings (enterocytes) through which the nutrients can enter the bloodstream.

Conversely, when the intestines are full their walls are stretched, which facilitates access for nutrients to be absorbed and then move into the bloodstream. The intestines are teeming with healthy and abundant microorganisms that encourage the absorption of nutrients.

☞ Good to Know

Efficient absorption of nutrients at the intestinal level is fundamental for good health. In this way the body benefits fully from the nutrients supplied by food.

THE ABILITY TO SYNTHESIZE VITAMINS AND OTHER NUTRIENTS

Vitamins and amino acids are generally recognized as essential for health. Because the body is not able to produce these substances itself, it is absolutely necessary that they be supplied to it. However, recent studies have shown that the intestinal microbiota, thanks to its high enzyme production, is capable of synthesizing some of these nutrients.

The nutrients that the intestinal microbiota can produce are:

> Vitamin B_{12}
> Vitamin B_1 (thiamine)
> Vitamin B_6
> Vitamin B_9 (folic acid)
> Vitamin PP (niacin)
> Vitamin N (biotin)
> Vitamin K
> Various amino acids

⚠ Take Note!

Nutrients that are synthesized by the intestinal microorganisms cannot cover all the body's needs by themselves. However, they are a useful supplement for people with strong and active intestinal flora.

ANTITOXIC FUNCTION

Countless toxic substances can find their way into a living organism and compromise its health. When one succeeds, it attacks and injures or destroys the cells of this organism, resulting in functional diseases with lesions that in some cases can even lead to death.

Intestinal microorganisms do not escape from this threat. Tiny as they are, they are still living beings that can be injured or destroyed by the action of certain poisons. They are not, however, defenseless. Like all living things, they can fight back against the attack. They do this primarily with the help of enzymes they manufacture themselves. These enzymes will neutralize the poisons by rendering them inoperative or breaking them down into simpler elements that have no dangerous properties. These elements are then either eliminated in this state or reabsorbed into the bloodstream to be used by the body.

The microorganisms of the intestine are very vulnerable to poisoning. The foods we eat today often carry toxic substances (herbicides, pesticides, food additives, poisons created by pollution, and so forth) with them into the body. The bacteria that live in our intestines are therefore the first to confront them. In addition, these bacteria share a limited living space with trillions of other individual microorganisms, each of which produces wastes that are partially toxic. In order to survive, the intestinal microorganisms must be capable of neutralizing these poisons.

🖐 Good to Know

Thanks to their large numbers, intestinal microorganisms perform an enormous amount of detoxification work. This work is estimated to be on a par with that of the liver, which is known to be the most powerful organ in the body when it comes to detoxification. Intestinal microorganisms, therefore, offer the body "a second liver" so that it can clean and purify itself.

When intestinal bacteria neutralize toxic substances it is self-protection, rather than an effort to rescue the human being, but we benefit from their efforts. By protecting themselves against attacks, they are also helping us since the poisons (or at least a portion of them) that would otherwise be able to make us sick are neutralized before they have a chance to harm us.

INTESTINAL TRANSIT FUNCTION

Sometimes the system can get clogged. Many people suffer from more or less severe constipation because their intestines are sluggish.

A number of different conditions must be in effect for the intestinal transit to proceed properly and at optimal speed. Some of them are common knowledge; for example, the intestines must get enough roughage and water. Others are less familiar but equally important, including having a healthy and balanced intestinal microbiota. There are a variety of ways in which intestinal bacteria normalize the intestinal transit.

Action on the Digestive Level

The primary purpose of peristaltic contractions is to move the alimentary bolus forward through the entire length (about twenty-five feet) of the intestines, and it is designed in a very intelligent way. If foods have not been fully digested within a particular part of the intestine, they will not be pushed further through the passage; the peristaltic movements slow to allow transformation of the food to be completed. However, by breaking foods down into small particles, the intestinal microorganisms encourage these transformations and remove the need for slowing of the peristaltic contractions. In this way the peristaltic movements are not hindered but supported.

Preparation of the Stool

Food wastes that remain after the digestive process has completed its work and the absorption of all the nutrients has taken place must be converted into a homogeneous bulk that is evenly moist and has a soft consistency. When the preparatory work has been entirely completed, stools like this are very easy for the body to eliminate. This job of transforming food remnants into stools is the responsibility of the intestinal microorganisms, especially those of the colon. When the microbiota is healthy with abundant microorganisms, the preparation of the stool is quick and transit is easy.

Production of Lactic Acid

The peristaltic muscles will only contract if they are stimulated. There are nerves scattered throughout the intestinal walls that give them the necessary impulses. One part of the stimulation results from the friction of dietary fibers against the intestinal walls, and another from the expansion of these walls when the intestine is full of food. But peristalsis can also be triggered by "stimulating" substances such as, among others, lactic acid, which is a byproduct of the activity of fermentation. This acid stimulates the nerve endings of the peristaltic muscles, thus encouraging intestinal transit.

Stimulation of the Production of Intestinal Mucus

When intestinal microorganisms come into contact with the mucous membranes of the intestinal walls, they have a slightly irritating effect. In order to mitigate this effect, the mucous membranes secrete a protective mucus with an oily consistency that encourages the stools to slip easily along the intestinal walls. This mucus acts in a way that is identical to that of oil in an engine. In fact, just as a motor can't function properly without enough oil to act as a lubricant, the intestines can only push the substances they contain through them if there is enough mucus.

? Did You Know?

The liver secretes bile that provides additional lubrication in the intestines.

▰ What We've Learned

The intestinal microbiota includes two major categories of microorganisms: the bacteria of fermentation and the bacteria of putrefaction. The microbiota has numerous duties: it plays a role in digestion, encourages absorption of nutrients, manufactures vitamins and amino acids, neutralizes toxins, and stimulates the intestinal transit.

3

Intestinal Flora
and Immune Defenses

Another role played by the microbiota is its contribution to the body's defense system. Much has been said about the bone marrow, the spleen, and the lymph glands as the primary organs of the immune system, but intestinal microorganisms are no less important. Moreover, the microbiota acts very efficiently and effectively to protect the body against microbial attacks. Its action is twofold:

- It kills microbes coming from outside the body.
- It stimulates the immune system to perform the same task.

BARRIER EFFECT

A subtle balance is maintained among the sizes of the various populations of intestinal microorganisms, the surfaces of the territories they occupy, the parts of the intestines they colonize, and the parts of foods to which they lay claim. This balance is not one that foreign microbe invaders can easily disrupt. It is difficult for these invaders to establish themselves in the intestines and multiply there because all the residential possibilities have already been exploited so fully. The living space they require in order to develop is unavailable and they lack nutrients. This is how, through its presence alone, the microbiota acts as a barrier against pathogenic bacteria. It prevents them from unleashing infections in the intestines or other parts of the body. This barrier effect can be total (extreme), in which case the newcomers have no possibility of gaining any kind of foothold; or partial (accessible), when it allows some bacteria to establish themselves but in numbers too insignificant to represent any kind of health threat. In the event there is an imbalance of the intestinal microorganisms, the barrier effect can be clearly insufficient. In this case there is no obstacle to pathogenic bacteria establishing themselves and multiplying, which eventually leads to an infection.

? Did You Know?

The destruction of bacteria by antibiotics often extends to the intestinal flora. When the flora suffer huge population losses, it makes living space available to other microorganisms. Because the barrier effect has vanished, pathogenic microbes can now move into these spaces. By multiplying, they are often the source of numerous infections.

ANTIBIOTIC EFFECT

The intestines are living environments for all the bacteria of the intestinal flora, and they need this environment in order to survive. This is why not even a single microorganism is ready to surrender space to invaders. They battle these invaders and seek to destroy them by releasing aggressive toxic substances. These substances are well known because certain ones are used in healing therapies: they are antibiotics.

This is how intestinal microorganisms defeat a portion of the pathogenic microbes that enter the body, thereby preventing them from attacking us. But this can only happen when the intestinal flora is healthy.

STIMULATION
OF LYMPHOCYTE PRODUCTION

The intestinal flora also takes part in the defense of the body by stimulating the production of the little "soldiers" of the immune system otherwise known as lymphocytes.

? Did You Know?

Of all the lymphocytes produced by the body to recognize and attack invading bacteria and toxins, 50 percent are in the digestive tract.

The composition of the intestinal flora is ever changing because it varies based on the arrival of microorganisms—both harmful and beneficial—that come from outside the body. The immune system is therefore obliged to be constantly monitoring what microbes are entering the intestines. It can do this thanks to plasmocytes and Peyer's patches.

Plasmocytes are isolated cells in the tissues located at regular intervals in the lower half of the small intestine (the ileum). They resemble T lymphocytes and B lymphocytes and, like them, they have the ability to detect dangerous microorganisms and analyze their characteristics. Using the information gained from this analysis, they then produce substances that can neutralize and destroy these invaders: immunoglobulins, also called antibodies. They have the ability to kill bacteria, or to prevent them from multiplying or attaching themselves to the walls of the intestines (thus ensuring they will be transported out of the body with the stools).

Peyer's patches—small masses of lymphatic tissue—are spread throughout the ileum region of the small intestine. They are cell clusters in the mucous membrane, the majority of which are B lymphocytes or B cells. Like plasmocytes, Peyer's patches also produce antibodies but in much larger numbers.

In this way the intestinal flora become more diverse due to different kinds of bacteria received from outside the body, causing greater variety in the kind of antibodies the microbiota produces. As a result the body has a larger arsenal of antibodies it can use to defend itself against any infections that arise.

REINFORCEMENT
OF THE IMMUNE SYSTEM

Abundant intestinal flora offers another important benefit to the immune system. The strong demand placed on the plasmocytes and Peyer's patches not only makes them stronger and therefore capable of producing more antibodies, it also ensures that as they multiply they increase the number of cells that are producing antibodies, which further strengthens the body's defenses. This aligns with the law of nature that "the function creates the organ." In other words, the greater the demand that is placed upon an organ, the stronger and more effective it will become at performing its functions. In this way, countless antibodies are prepared to go into action not only in the intestines but also, if necessary, in other parts of the body that are being attacked by pathogenic microorganisms. Indeed, the bloodstream can easily transport them throughout the body.

PRACTICAL APPLICATION

**Food Sterilization
and Lowered Immunity**

Given that the immune system is kept active and effective thanks to its multiple contacts with external bacteria and other microorganisms, it is a mistake to try to sterilize all our foods in order to avoid infection. This process actually reduces the effectiveness of the immune system by reducing the number of antibodies it has available.

ANTI-INFLAMMATORY ACTION

The anti-infective function of the intestinal flora is accompanied by an anti-inflammatory effect. Diseases characterized by inflammation are in fact caused by attacks on the tissues, whether the culprits are bacteria or toxic substances. As it happens, intestinal bacteria have a strong ability to oppose both of these causes of inflammation, thanks to their antibiotic and antitoxic functions. Their action, therefore, has an anti-inflammatory effect.

A more specific action combines with this general effect. Some intestinal microorganisms appear to secrete anti-inflammatory substances, for it has been observed that when this strain of microorganism diminishes below its normal numbers, an inflammatory disease can develop more easily. This is the case with Crohn's disease, for example. Its characteristic symptoms are inflammation of the intestinal mucous membranes, abdominal pain, and diarrhea. The populations of *Faecalibacterium* and *Firmicutes* are much smaller in those who are suffering from this disease than in people who are not. Health researchers have concluded from this that if these intestinal bacteria are present in sufficient number, one or more substances they release prevents the intestinal mucous membranes from becoming inflamed, and therefore can be labeled as anti-inflammatory substances.

🎓 What We've Learned

The intestinal flora plays a fundamental role in the body's immune system:

- Its presence prevents pathogenic bacteria from establishing themselves in the intestines (the barrier effect).

- It produces antibiotic substances that kill dangerous bacteria.

- It stimulates the production of lymphocytes and antibodies.

- Its antitoxic and antibiotic properties make its action anti-inflammatory.

4

Enemies of
the Intestinal Flora

Enemies of the intestinal flora are factors that sharply reduce the population of microorganisms and thus compromise our health. Their destructive effect is not uniform across all the different kinds of intestinal bacteria but can have a very strong effect on some intestinal microorganisms and a very weak or no effect whatsoever on others. The bacteria that are most often affected are generally those of fermentation that populate the small intestine and the beginning of the colon. The bacteria of putrefaction that live in the terminus of the colon are much less affected. Normally the bacteria of fermentation and those of putrefaction are balanced. When this balance is disrupted, a number of health problems can arise that will be described in this chapter.

The intestinal flora performs a number of functions that are very useful for the body: digestion, detoxification, immune system support, and so on. The effectiveness of the work it does is dependent, however, on the quantity of microorganisms in the intestinal flora. When this flora is abundant and strong, its work is more powerful than when it is reduced in number and weak. Consequently, factors that reduce the number of intestinal microorganisms have an adverse effect. The various functions that are carried out by the flora—functions the body depends on—become lethargic and less effective.

? Did You Know?

The intestinal flora has various enemies that can weaken it. Lack of dietary fiber and use of antibiotics are the most dangerous.

Let's first take a look at the identities of these enemies of the intestinal flora. These enemies have such a direct connection with our lifestyle that it's very easy for us to take steps to neutralize them.

LACK OF FIBER

Every living thing requires a specific kind of food: lions eat meat, cows eat grass, and so forth. The food required by the bacteria of fermentation in our intestinal flora is the fiber in our human diet. It should be noted that fiber is a choice food for the bacteria of fermentation and not for those of putrefaction because usually fiber has already been digested when the food arrives in the region where this bacteria lives—the end of the colon. The bacteria of putrefaction feed on the proteins, carbohydrates, and lipids that have not been completely digested in the upper regions of the digestive tract.

If the bacteria of fermentation receive adequate fiber, they will be healthy and strong, and they will multiply easily. The production of new bacteria increases and easily compensates for the microorganisms continually being killed by other bacteria or by toxins, or being carried away by stool.

When fiber intake is low, on the other hand, the quantity of bacteria of fermentation in the intestinal flora will also shrink to smaller proportions. In fact, the quantity of food always determines the size of the population that depends on it. Small quantities of fiber can feed only a small number of bacteria, so the population of bacteria of fermentation will shrink. The diminished population will be weakened and thus more vulnerable to attack, the consequence of which is a further reduction of their numbers.

The three dietary fibers that are the preferred foods of the flora of fermentation are all of plant origin: mucilaginous substances (found in, for example, okra and flax seeds), pectins (found in, for example, apples and guavas), and oligosaccharides (found in legumes, nuts, and so on). Consequently, individuals who do not eat enough plant foods—fruits, vegetables, grains, nuts, and beans—have a deficiency of fiber. This is common in diets that are poor in salad greens, both raw and cooked vegetables, nuts (almonds, hazelnuts), and whole grains.

✚ Tips and Tricks

Foods that are high in fiber should be eaten several times a day. Grains in particular should be consumed in their whole form (whole grain bread and pasta, unrefined brown rice) because refined grains (white flour bread and pasta) contain very little fiber.

The importance of fiber for the fermentation flora stems from the fact that this flora depends entirely on the fibers from food to work and survive. An intake of sufficient fiber is therefore a key factor in the health of the intestinal flora and consequently our overall health.

DEHYDRATION

The environment of the intestines is a liquid environment. The foods that travel through it do so in the form of a puree that is created thanks to the secretion of some seven quarts of digestive juices every day.

The intestinal microorganisms need this liquid environment in order to thrive. Any substantial reduction of the amount of liquid in the intestines will be harmful to them and their numbers will diminish. This is the case for all those people who do not drink the two to two and a half quarts of liquid (water, herbal teas, and so on) that the body needs daily and who eat only a small amount of juicy fruits and vegetables. The organic tissues will suffer from a deficiency of fluid and steal what they need from the intestines. Stools will become drier and harder to expel, leading to constipation and a reduction of bacteria populations in the microbiota.

? Did You Know?

Every day the body secretes more than a quart of saliva, a quart and a half of gastric juices, three-quarters of a quart of pancreatic fluids and of bile, and more than three quarts of intestinal juices.

OVERDOING RAW VEGETABLES

Raw fruits and vegetables are beneficial to our health because they are high in vitamins, minerals, trace elements, and enzymes. It is therefore recommended that everyone eat a good amount of them on a regular basis. Some people take this advice too far and eat too many raw foods on a daily basis.

The fibers these foods provide are certainly choice fare for the intestinal flora. Eaten in excess, however, fiber has the effect of roughly scraping the intestinal mucous membranes, which overly stimulates the peristaltic movements. The rhythm of the intestinal transit is speeded up and the contents of the intestines are pushed through too vigorously, carrying the intestinal bacteria toward the lower end of the intestines. This causes them to have greater difficulty in attaching to the walls of the intestines, which they need in order to establish themselves and multiply. The size of the intestinal flora shrinks in numbers of bacteria and the remaining bacteria have trouble restoring the flora to its former size.

PRACTICAL APPLICATION

Avoiding Fiber Irritation

- The irritation hazard does not exist for cooked fruits and vegetables, as the fibers they contain have been softened by cooking and are consequently less stimulating.
- Large quantities of vegetable juices and fruit juices don't irritate the intestinal walls, as juices contain a minimum amount of fiber, if any.

The wisest path for each individual is to discover the best-suited proportions of cooked to raw foods. In this way people can nourish their unique balance of intestinal flora without causing harm by overdoing it.

EXCESS WHITE FLOUR, WHITE BREAD, WHITE RICE, AND SO ON

Refinement of cereal grains strips away the outer layers of these grains, which is where their fibers are primarily located. Refined grains are not completely devoid of fiber but they contain a great deal less roughage than whole grains. A person who eats white rice and bread and pasta made from refined flour will have poorly fed intestinal flora that may not be adequate to ensure good digestive health.

OVEREATING OF FATS

The digestive juice responsible for the digestion of fats is the bile secreted by the liver. When someone eats a diet rich in high-fat foods—butter, cream, cheese, sausage, fried foods, pastries, and so forth—it puts a lot of demand on the liver. The bile secreted by the liver is alkaline, so when the quantity increases, bile can alkalize the small intestine. This stops the bacteria of fermentation from developing properly because they require an environment that is slightly acidic. Their numbers will drop as a result.

OVEREATING OF MEAT AND ANIMAL PROTEINS

Meat does contain fiber but it is not the same fiber as that found in vegetables, which are the only fibers that the bacteria of fermentation can use as a food supply. There is absolutely no fiber content in cheese and eggs. Diets that consist in large part of meat, cheese, and eggs are therefore not contributing anything significant to feeding and maintaining the bacteria of fermentation.

ALCOHOL

Excessive alcohol is known to have a drying effect that eventually will lead to hardening of the gastric and intestinal mucous membrane cells. The same effect takes place on the bacteria of the intestinal flora, as they are also cells, leading to an overall weakening of the intestinal flora.

PURGES

The daily evacuation of stools quite naturally leads to the elimination of a certain quantity of the bacteria that reside in the intestines. These are in the alimentary bolus, which inevitably leads to their departure from the body when this bolus is expelled (in the form of stools). This loss of bacteria is normally compensated for by the production of new bacteria by the resident intestinal flora.

However, the loss of bacteria is much greater when the system is flushed with a purge, or purgative, which acts like a laxative but in a much more intense way. The purpose of a purge is to energetically empty the intestine of its contents, but it doesn't discriminate. When the purge carries out a large amount of very fluid fecal matter, it also washes away a large number of intestinal bacteria. The microbiota will be temporarily weakened after a purge. Purges also drive the fermentation bacteria into the lower intestine, which is an acidic environment in which they can't survive.

While an occasional castor oil or saline purge when necessary is not harmful, purges should not be overused. (See my book *Freedom from Constipation,* Rochester, Vt.: Healing Arts Press, 2017, 168–70.)

ANTIBIOTICS

Antibiotics are among the most often prescribed medications, and they are another major enemy of the intestinal flora. Their role is to kill living organisms that attack the body, but they don't necessarily discriminate. The living organisms they target are pathogenic microbes, but in the process antibiotics also kill other microorganisms. There are more than one hundred types of antibiotics and some cause more damage to the intestinal flora than others, and in different ways. Varying factors need to be taken into account.

? Did You Know?

The deleterious effect of antibiotics can be quick and powerful. Although beneficial against pathogens, some reduce the intestinal flora to half its former size in five to seven days, and their harmful effects can be felt for three to six months.

Range of Activity

Some antibiotics are able to kill a number of different kinds of disease-causing bacteria; they are known as broad-spectrum antibiotics because of the range of their activity. Other antibiotics have an effect on only one kind of bacteria or another, and they are known as narrow-spectrum antibiotics. Because they are less specialized, antibiotics with a broad spectrum of activity attack the characteristics that are common to many different strains of bacteria. These kinds of antibiotics more easily damage the bacteria of the intestinal flora.

Length of Treatment

Antibiotics can work more or less quickly depending on the type and whether the troublesome bacteria are resistant to them. During a short course, some microorganisms that could be vulnerable may escape damage due to the limited time they are in contact with the antibiotic. This means that the damage caused to the intestinal flora is limited in scope.

Conversely, during a longer period of treatment contact is prolonged. The antibiotic is more thorough and effective, but it also destroys many intestinal microorganisms.

Repetition of Treatment

Some intestinal bacteria always manage to survive initial contact with an antibiotic they are vulnerable to, but this contact still leaves them in a weakened state and they are unable to resist if a new treatment follows the first one too closely.

PRACTICAL APPLICATION
....
**Avoiding Destruction of
the Intestinal Flora during Infections**

Antibiotics that are created in a laboratory are not the only ones in existence. Numerous medicinal plants, such as thyme, eucalyptus, lapacho (*pau d'arco*), and so on also have antibiotic properties and do not kill intestinal flora. For more on this subject I suggest interested readers consult my book on natural antibiotics (*Natural Antibiotics and Antivirals,* Rochester, Vt.: Healing Arts Press, 2018).

CHEMOTHERAPY

Chemotherapy, a healing technique for cancer, uses toxic chemical substances to stop cancerous cells from growing and multiplying, and this eventually kills them. Some of the intestinal microorganisms that come into contact with these substances are also vulnerable to them and die. The balance is then disrupted, causing dysbiosis. Conversely, scientists are now finding that regulating gut bacteria can diminish side effects of chemotherapy, which can be explained by the antitoxic function of the intestinal flora.

🎓 What We've Learned

The intestinal flora has enemies that can weaken or destroy it:

- A diet low in fruits, vegetables, and whole grain foods does not supply the intestinal flora with the fiber it needs to feed itself.
- Overconsumption of proteins, white sugar, and fats causes harmful changes to the environment needed by the intestinal bacteria so that it can survive and thrive.
- Antibiotics kill intestinal flora.
- Excessive use of purgatives washes away a large amount of intestinal bacteria.

5

Intestinal
Flora Imbalance
and Disease

The enemies of the intestinal flora reduce the number of microorganisms of fermentation. This circumstance is already harmful enough on its own, but another one accompanies it: an imbalance between the populations of the fermentation bacteria and the putrefaction bacteria can also pose a grave threat to overall physical health. It is a fact that many different health disorders originate from unbalanced intestinal flora, or dysbiosis.

IMBALANCE IN
THE INTESTINAL FLORA

Together the flora of fermentation and the flora of putrefaction make up the intestinal microbiota. The quality of this flora is dependent on the balance between these two kinds of bacteria. There are more bacteria of fermentation, which makes perfect sense as these bacteria colonize a much larger part of the intestines: the entire small intestine (sixteen feet) and a large part of the colon (a little more than three feet), versus the descending colon alone (one and a half feet) for bacteria of putrefaction.

We still discuss this in terms of a balance between the two flora—the state that exists when each type occupies its portion of the intestines without invading the territory of the other. When these circumstances are in place, the intestinal flora consists of 85 percent flora of fermentation and 15 percent flora of putrefaction. These are the ideal proportions for a healthy microbiota. Any change in these proportions is, conversely, a sign of imbalance and an indication that the microbiota is not healthy. Such changes are caused by the enemies of the intestinal flora that were discussed in the preceding chapter.

Let's take a look at how diet, for example, can have a destabilizing effect on the intestinal flora and upset its balance. In order to survive, intestinal bacteria depend on the foods we eat, because they supply this bacteria with the required nutrients. When the nutrients they need are available to them in ample supply, their numbers increase. The opposite occurs when they are receiving a reduced quantity of nutrients: the number of bacteria in the microbiota also diminishes.

However, the majority of people today eat a diet that is lacking in fruits, vegetables, and whole grains. It therefore contains very little of the fiber that bacteria of fermentation require in order to propagate. On the contrary, the typical modern diet is high in meats and a variety of other proteins, foods that are the select diet for bacteria of putrefaction. The net result of this diet is to reduce the quantity of fermentation flora while increasing that of putrefaction flora. In drastic cases the proportions of the two different types of flora can become the exact opposite of what they should be.

When this kind of reversal takes place, the microbes of putrefaction can become too abundant to be confined in the descending colon. In order to survive, this population expands its living space in the only direction it can: higher in the intestine, outside of its normal territory into the transverse colon and the ascending colon. This kind of expansion is all too possible and is made all the easier when the flora of fermentation that normally colonize these parts of the digestive tract are already reduced in number and scattered due to the same imbalance. They therefore no longer pose any obstacle to the advance of the bacteria of putrefaction. The barrier effect has been eliminated. Furthermore, because the quantity of fermentation flora has been reduced, the acidity it produced—and which served as another barrier to the bacteria of putrefaction—no longer exists. The environment is more alkaline, which also encourages the invasion of bacteria of putrefaction that thrive in this kind of environment.

The imbalance of the intestinal flora that I have just described that was caused by a lack of fiber in the diet can also occur in connection with antibiotics and other enemies of the intestinal flora. All the enemies of the intestinal flora have the effect of disrupting the balance between bacteria of fermentation and of putrefaction. Whether they reduce the population of the fermentation flora (the most common case) or increase the numbers of putrefaction flora (with an excess of proteins, fats, or other substances), the final result every time is an imbalance that prevents the intestinal flora from functioning properly. There are a number of disorders that can arise from this unbalanced state. The principal ones are the following:

INDIGESTION

Good digestion is the result of the combined activity of the digestive juices and the intestinal flora. If the participation of one of these actors is missing or is only partially performed, which is the case when the intestinal flora is flawed, digestion is compromised. The poorly digested foods stagnate in the digestive tract. The congested state this causes creates various symptoms of indigestion: abdominal sensitivity to pressure, pain, nausea, vomiting, a general sense of malaise, headaches, and so forth.

GAS AND BLOATING

The production of gas is a normal phenomenon during the digestive process. It is minimal however, for it is primarily caused by all the activity of the bacteria of putrefaction that are normally confined to the descending colon. In this case the gases are easily transported in a non-gaseous form by the bloodstream and expelled through the respiratory tract. This process normally takes place without anyone noticing.

When there is an imbalance of the intestinal flora and putrefaction bacteria invade the entire length of the colon and the end of the small intestine, their increased numbers produce more gas. If the amount of gas to be expelled surpasses the body's ability to expel it, the gas lies stagnant in the intestines, causing the swollen sensation of being bloated. The gas can also be expelled through the lower end of the intestines, which is the source of problems with flatulence.

The odor of the gas comes first and foremost from the putrefaction of proteins. The transformation of proteins in the colon produces phenols and skatole, which are particularly malodorous substances. The greater the disruption to the flora, which translates into a larger preponderance of the bacteria of putrefaction, the more unpleasant the odor.

? Did You Know?

The odorless gases that are created from a weakness of the intestinal flora are not caused by proteins but by carbohydrates (white sugar, white bread, sweets and pasta made from refined flour, and so on).

WHITE TONGUE, COATED MOUTH

Many people wake up in the morning with a white-coated tongue and mouth. This can happen when an increased amount of putrefaction flora develops, because it leads to a significant increase in the production of toxic substances (in addition to the gas we just discussed above).

Once they have been absorbed into the bloodstream, toxic substances are transported to the liver to be neutralized. However, if the amount of toxins is too high, it may exceed the liver's ability to process. In this case the bloodstream carries them further and they spread throughout the body, which then attempts to eliminate them. One of the body's methods of elimination is through the mucous membranes of the digestive system. This is how the tongue can become saturated with wastes and turn white. When this is the case the tongue is sometimes described as being "coated." The same is true for the mouth. These disorders disappear once the natural balance of intestinal flora is restored.

? Did You Know?

Hippocrates (460–377 BCE), the Father of Medicine, said, "All illnesses start in the intestines," thereby indirectly emphasizing the importance of the intestinal flora.

DIARRHEA

The purpose of the various processes of digestion is to reduce the foods we ingest into very tiny particles so that our intestines can absorb nutrients and pass them on to other parts of our bodies. As long as they have not yet reached this stage, fragments of food in the intestines are regarded by our physical organism as foreign bodies. This is the case when the intestinal flora is deficient, as it no longer performs its proper role in the digestive process. The poorly digested food fragments irritate the walls of the intestines and cause them to become inflamed. The intestines then try to get rid of these fragments as quickly as possible, which they do by releasing more mucus in order to reduce their concentration. One consequence of this increased mucus production is that the stools will be made more liquid and therefore easier to eliminate. The rapid and repeated elimination of soft and watery stools that results is what we call diarrhea.

⚠ Take Note!

One side effect of antibiotics, diarrhea, is very common. This occurs because these drugs weaken the intestinal flora's ability to digest the foods we eat.

When incidents of diarrhea are of short duration, they may be the result of eating a meal that is too rich, and unrelated to the intestinal flora. However, when diarrhea is repeated over a span of time with watery and shapeless stools, its cause is almost certainly a deficiency of the intestinal flora.

PRACTICAL APPLICATION
....
Causes of Overly Rapid Intestinal Transit

An intestinal transit that takes place too rapidly can be recognized by two or three liquid stools rather than one stool of proper solid consistency. In addition to being caused by excessive ingestion of raw foods, it can also be attributed to:

- Stress
- Drinking too much coffee or ingesting too many other stimulants
- Overeating and indigestible food mixtures (e.g., fruits with starches), which lead to poor digestion and the production of irritating substances, such as indole and skatole

---

FOOD ALLERGIES

When the intestinal flora remains out of balance for a long time, the quantity of toxic substances being produced by the flora of putrefaction starts to regularly get into the bloodstream. This constantly triggers a response from the immune system. If the situation persists, the immune system eventually becomes hypersensitive and hyperreactive. Because of this mal-function, it starts to trigger excessively strong defense reactions that also target friendly food substances. These reactions that the body uses to defend itself are essentially allergic reactions. They can manifest as digestive tract spasms (abdominal pains), respiratory tract spasms (coughs, asthma), and in the form of skin rashes (hives, eczema).

☞ Good to Know

In the event of food allergies, the body's defense reactions are not evidence of any actual danger in the food but reveal rather a dysfunction of the immune system—a dysfunction created by a deficiency of intestinal flora and of the mucous membranes.

INTESTINAL POROSITY
AND AUTOINTOXICATION

When the intestinal flora does not properly disintegrate foods into fragments small enough to be usable by the body and does not neutralize wastes, poisons, and toxins, the large food mol-ecules and poisons attack the walls of the intestine. Over the long term this causes microlesions, which make the intestines porous.

When the intestinal mucous membranes become porous it can be extremely detrimental to health, as this allows toxins and poisons to permeate the walls, enter the blood-stream, and travel to any spot in the body. This surreptitious poisoning causes the cellular terrain to deteriorate, which is the cause of a large number of health disorders and diseases.

? Did You Know?

The accumulation of toxic substances in the body's cellular terrain is, according to natural medicine, the root cause of most of our illnesses.

AUTOIMMUNE DISEASES

The toxins and other harmful substances produced by the pathogenic bacteria of the intestinal flora do not pose any threat to the body when the flora is in balance. These pathogenic microorganisms are few in number and the quantity of poisons they produce is so small that it can easily be neutralized by other intestinal bacteria. This situation changes when the intestinal flora is weakened and the barrier effect is no longer in force against the disease-causing bacteria. The harmful bacteria increases radically, which increases the quantity of other harmful substances, such as acetaldehyde, which can alter the structure of some of the body's proteins.

The immune system now detects cells in the organic tissues that are formed from different proteins from those of the rest of the body. It naturally considers them as foreign and therefore dangerous, which requires a defensive reaction on its part. The immune system then sends lymphocytes to destroy them, but in so doing, the body is fighting against itself. It is self-destructing.

The autoimmune diseases that result can also affect the intestines (celiac disease, Crohn's disease, hemorrhagic rectal colitis, and so on), muscles (myasthenia), nerves (multiple sclerosis), skin (psoriasis, piebald skin, and so forth), and other parts of the body.

MENTAL DISORDERS

When the intestinal flora becomes imbalanced and the bacteria of putrefaction multiply and increase production of noxious toxins, they are carried throughout the body and disrupt the functioning of many organs, including the nervous system and the brain. This can interfere with our mental balance and the way we feel about life and approach it, leading some people to suffer from anxiety, fear, or depression.

VARIOUS INFECTIOUS DISEASES

An imbalance of the intestinal flora provides a favorable incubator for infectious diseases. When the barrier effect is no longer fully active, some microorganisms start to multiply and their harmful effects on the body are soon fully apparent.

The microbes responsible for infections are of various strains and have different origins. There are several possible primary causes:

External Pathogenic Microorganisms

A harmful microorganism enters the body by means of food or drink. If the intestinal flora is deficient, it doesn't have to stand up to a very large population or stronger strain of bacteria. This noxious microbe easily finds a space to establish itself where it can find enough of the food it needs. There it multiplies and when its population has grown sufficiently, it unleashes an infection.

⊕ Tips and Tricks

Travelers' diarrhea, a type of gastroenteritis that strikes many tourists when they visit tropical countries, afflicts only travelers whose intestinal flora is weak.

Internal Pathogenic Microorganisms

Not all the microorganisms that make us sick come from outside the body. Some are already present in our body's intestinal flora, but in numbers too small to pose any danger to our health. The situation changes when the intestinal flora falls out of balance and enters a weakened state. Because they are no longer hindered by the barrier effect, these noxious strains of bacteria begin to multiply and start moving to other regions of the body, where they cause this or that organ to become ill.

Staphylococci and *Streptococci* are bacteria found almost everywhere in our natural environment (water, dirt) but also reside in small numbers in our intestines. Most of the time when they make us ill it is because they have entered our respiratory tract or an open wound from outside the body. However, in some people whose intestinal flora has been weakened it is caused by the *Staphylococci* and *Streptococci* that already reside in the intestinal flora. When they are allowed to multiply because the flora is no longer functioning properly, they can trigger various infections. These infections can take a variety of forms depending on their location: enteritis, urinary infections, angina, nasopharyngitis, pneumonia, boils, abscesses, impetigo, arteritis, endocarditis, meningitis, blood poisoning, and so on.

Among the other pathological bacteria normally present in the intestinal flora we have E. coli (enteritis and cystitis); *Klebsiella* (infections that can affect the respiratory tract, digestive tract, and urogenital system); shigella (dysentery), salmonella (typhoid), and so forth.

As can be easily seen, the infections that these different strains of bacteria cause are not limited to the intestines but travel easily around the body. This can take the form of bacteria going back through the digestive system to reach the upper respiratory tract or colonizing the genital and urinary tract. Some of them can also escape from the intestines through microlesions in the intestinal walls to the bloodstream, which then carries them to other parts of the body.

☝ Good to Know

Eighty percent of all cases of cystitis are triggered by the E. coli bacteria. *Escherichia coli* is a regular guest of our intestines because it forms part of the intestinal flora. When the intestinal flora is out of balance and weakened, these bacteria multiply and migrate into the urinary tract, triggering a painful infection.

Nonpathogenic Internal Microorganisms

Numerous microorganisms of the microbiota are benign on their own under normal circumstances—when they are confined to an organ that can easily support their presence and their numbers remain sufficiently small. However, when they multiply and migrate to other organs that are unable to tolerate their presence, these microorganisms stop being benign and become quite detrimental to our health.

This is the case, for example, with *Candida albicans,* a fungus, or more specifically a yeast that is a normal resident of the intestines. Normally its population remains quite small and it plays an insignificant role in physiological function. It would probably have remained completely unknown to the general public if the destruction of intestinal flora by excessive use of antibiotics had not given it the means to multiply out of proportion. When overgrowth happens, this yeast colonizes the digestive tract and then migrates into the respiratory tract, the urogenital system, and the skin, where it causes infections and fungal growth. *Candida* is also a factor in chronic fatigue, hormonal disorders, and immune system dysfunction.

The many different toxins it releases (around eighty, all told) can also have a deleterious effect on the nervous system. This can cause nerve and emotional disorders such as anxiety, irritability, fear, mood swings, lack of concentration, and impaired memory.

INFLAMMATORY DISEASES

Some of the substances produced by the intestinal flora can be irritating and invasive to our tissues, leading to inflammation.

When there is an imbalance in the intestinal flora, the production of substances that cause inflammation is greatly increased. Their contact with the intestinal mucous membranes over a long period of time makes the gut susceptible to a variety of disorders characterized by inflammation, such as irritable bowel syndrome, enteritis, colitis, and so forth.

Substances that have these inflammation-causing properties can also emigrate out of the intestines and travel into other regions of the body. In the urogenital system they can cause cystitis, urethritis, vaginitis, and so on. In the respiratory tract they can cause bronchitis. If they end up in the muscles they can cause lumbago and other disorders.

OBESITY

The kind of overeating that leads to obesity also causes the intestinal flora to go out of balance. This imbalance seems to encourage weight gain among people with that predisposition: substances released by certain strains of bacteria make it easier to store fat in the tissues. In addition, people who have imbalanced intestinal flora with minimal bacterial diversity gain weight more easily than those whose flora is balanced and varied.

🎓 What We've Learned

- Intestinal flora is said to be balanced and healthy when it consists of 85 percent flora of fermentation and 15 percent flora of putrefaction.
- When the numbers of bacteria of fermentation shrink, the population of the bacteria of putrefaction grows and invades the territory of the bacteria of fermentation. This imbalance engenders a variety of health disorders.
- The intestinal problems caused by an imbalance of the intestinal flora include indigestion, gas, bloating, diarrhea, and constipation.
- General disorders that can be attributed to disruption in the normal functioning of the intestinal flora are infections, inflammations, food allergies, autoimmune diseases, some mental disorders, and weight gain.

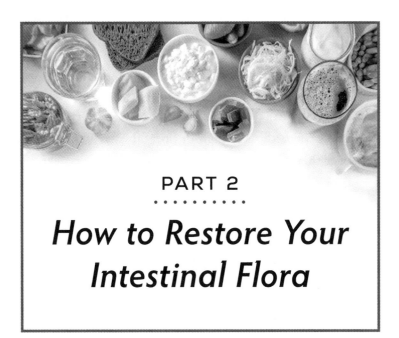

PART 2
. . . .
How to Restore Your Intestinal Flora

Three different complementary approaches are used to rebuild the flora of fermentation. When they are strong and healthy the bacteria of fermentation will easily multiply.

FIRST APPROACH

The first approach consists of feeding these bacteria well by consuming foods that are high in fiber, also called prebiotics. However, this slow process shows results only after a certain period of time. If there is a pressing need to make change quickly, proceed to the second approach.

SECOND APPROACH

This approach consists of implanting a large number of fermentation bacteria from outside the body into the intestines. This is done by means of probiotics, meaning foods or special preparations that contain a multitude of these bacteria. Instead of waiting for the bacteria that are present to multiply, this approach brings a large number directly into the body from outside. This increases the population and allows it to gradually return to its normal size.

THIRD APPROACH

This approach is indirect. It acts on the bacteria of putrefaction to decrease their numbers. In fact, any reduction in the size of the putrefaction bacteria population will encourage an increase in the fermentation population.

6

Feeding the Bacteria of Fermentation with Prebiotics

Prebiotics are dietary substances that consist of or contain a carbohydrate and encourage the activity and multiplication of the bacteria of fermentation. They come in the form of plant fiber that cannot be digested by human beings but can be digested by the fermentation bacteria, particularly those that reside in the lower part of the small intestine and in the ascending colon.

⚠ Take Note!

It is important not to confuse prebiotics for probiotics. Probiotics are bacteria with activity that is beneficial for our health. Prebiotics are the foods that nourish these bacteria.

TWO KINDS OF FIBER

Prebiotics are plant fibers, but this doesn't mean that all the fibers contained in the foods we eat are prebiotics, nor that foods high in fiber are necessarily a rich source of prebiotics. In fact, a distinction is made between two kinds of fibers.

Insoluble Fibers

Insoluble fibers are those fibers that form the protective husk of cereal grains (the pericarp or bran) or the substance that makes the plant structure stiff, such as the stem, for example. These fibers are in the form of cellulose. They are hard and coarse, and too much insoluble fiber irritates the intestinal walls.

Insoluble fibers are formed of chains of glucose that can include anywhere from 10,000 to 250,000 units. Because of their length and their insoluble nature, these fibers cannot be broken down into smaller particles, meaning they cannot be digested by the bacteria of fermentation. The bacteria cannot get any nourishment from these fibers, which is why insoluble fibers are not considered prebiotics. Their role in the intestines is to provide roughage that contributes to a healthy intestinal transit.

PRACTICAL APPLICATION

Roughage Has No Prebiotic Properties

Wheat and oat bran are recommended as roughage to fight against constipation, because they are both so high in fiber. They consist of 43 percent and 15 percent fiber respectively. Since the fiber they contain is insoluble, it has no prebiotic properties.

Soluble Fibers

These fibers are composed of short chains of glucose that consist of as few as two and no more than twenty units of glucose. The simple nature of these chains makes them easily digestible by the bacteria of fermentation. Furthermore, the soluble nature allows these bacteria to easily transform through the processes of hydrolysis and fermentation. Because soluble fibers can be used as food by the bacteria of fermentation, they are prebiotics. They are soft and consequently do not pose any threat of irritation to the intestines.

? Did You Know?

All plant foods contain soluble and insoluble fibers, but the proportions of each fiber vary from one food to the next.

THE DIFFERENT KINDS OF
SOLUBLE FIBERS

Soluble fibers are extremely small, which often means they are not visible to the naked eye. They are found in the skin of fruits and vegetables, but they can also appear in the flesh. They are also abundantly present in grains and beans. There are several kinds of these fibers.

Pectin

This is a mucilaginous substance present in many plant foods. Pectin is primarily known as a gelling agent for jams and jellies, since one of its characteristics is that it expands on contact with water. This allows it to form a solid mass that makes the jelly less liquid. A food that is well-known for having high pectin content is the apple.

Inulin (Fructan)

This substance has a composition close to that of starch, but its structure is much less complex. It consists of a blend of fructose and a variety of other simple sugars. Inulin can be found in many plants, but particularly in chicory roots and in the tubers of Jerusalem artichokes.

Fructooligosaccharides (FOS)

These carbohydrates are composed of fructose and other simple sugars, such as sucrose, lactose, and maltose. They are found in high amounts in chicory root and Jerusalem artichokes, as well as in beans, whole grains, and other plant foods.

Galactooligosaccharides (GOS)

These fibers consist of galactose in combination with other simple sugars. Galactooligosaccharides are the form in which plants store carbohydrates as a reserve fuel. This is why they are primarily found in the seeds of leguminous plants, seaweed-derived products, and root vegetables (beets, onions, Jerusalem artichokes, and so on).

NON-PLANT SOURCES OF PREBIOTICS

The newly created intestinal flora of a newborn baby is unable to feed itself on plant fibers as the baby is getting nourishment only through mother's milk, which does not contain any fiber. This flora will develop, however, thanks to the human milk oligosaccharides (HMO) or glycans in breast milk. The intestinal flora of babies who have been breastfed is consequently stronger and better balanced than that of formula-fed infants. Their digestion is easier and they have greater resistance to infections.

? Did You Know?

Galactooligosaccharides are found, in a slightly altered form, in breast milk. It contains nearly three ounces per quart.

Another source of prebiotics is cows' milk, which contains at least 0.17 ounce of carbohydrates per quart in the form of lactose. This is a bisaccharide that is made up of equal parts glucose and galactose—the same galactose that is found in GOS and HMO. This is how the digestion of lactose releases galactose that can then be used as a prebiotic for the intestinal bacteria.

Whey, a byproduct of milk, is rich in lactose and for this reason has long been used successfully to regenerate the intestinal flora. It is also high in amino acids and protein.

Sources of Prebiotics

Origin	Form	Source
Plant	Fibers	Fruits, vegetables, grains
Animal	Lactose, galactose	Whey, milk sugar

FOOD SOURCES OF PREBIOTICS

Prebiotics are found in a variety of sources, most of which are widely available.

Fruits

All fruits provide prebiotics that are useful for our intestinal flora, whether they are common to Europe and North America, like apples, pears, and grapes; or come from tropical regions: pineapple, papayas, bananas, and so on. These fruits can all be consumed fresh to enjoy their benefits, but they are just as helpful when dried. Dried fruits include dates, figs, raisins, apricots, prunes, mangoes, and many more.

Instructions for Use

Fruits are an ideal snack because they provide energy due to the carbohydrates they contain. They are able to raise the energy levels of the physical organism without demanding any great effort by the body, because they are easy to digest. They also make it easier to avoid eating bad sugars (such as those found in sodas or pastries) that place a much heavier demand on the digestive functions and add toxins.

EXAMPLES OF HEALTHY FRUIT SNACKS

- One or two fully ripened seasonal fruits, such as pears or persimmons
- A handful of dried fruits: dates, figs, or raisins, for example, with a couple of almonds
- Banana with almonds or almond butter
- A handful of mixed fruits and nuts
- A juiced fruit with pulp included (as juice or as part of a smoothie)

Fruits also make an appetizing and healthy dessert:

- Fruit salad
- Fruit compote
- Fruit tart

✪ Tips and Tricks

Fresh fruits consumed at the end of a meal are not tolerated by everyone. They can give some people gas and bloating. These people would be wiser to eat fruit as a snack between meals.

Vegetables

Vegetables that are high in fiber can also be helpful as prebiotics. Cooking vegetables can change the quality of these fibers, however, if they are cooked for too long or at too high a temperature. To ensure a sufficient intake of prebiotics from vegetables, it is recommended that most of them be eaten raw.

Instructions for Use

Vegetables can be eaten raw in the form of green salad, crudités (including shredded carrots or celery, or sliced tomatoes or cucumbers), mixed salad (salad greens combined with a variety of raw vegetables), juiced with pulp, or as vegetable sticks (carrots, cucumbers, peppers, turnip, with dip); cooked to taste; or simmered in homemade vegetable soup.

There are three foods in particular that should be presented in detail because they are not very common: chicory roots, dandelion roots, and Jerusalem artichokes.

✎ Chicory and Dandelion Roots

The roots of both these plants are exceptionally high in prebiotics: 64.6 percent for dried chicory root and 24.3 percent for dandelion root. However, neither of these plants falls into the range of commonly consumed foods. How are we supposed to eat them?

Instructions for use: Both these roots should be eaten raw. They can be dug up from the garden, but sometimes they can also be found in herb stores, in dried form. They therefore need to be rehydrated by letting them steep for a period of time in a bowl of water. Given their high concentration of fiber (in the form of FOS), there is no need to eat a lot of them at one time. About two teaspoons should be sufficient as a maintenance dose, with twice that much required in the case of severe imbalance of the intestinal flora. But look out, these roots have a bitter taste!

Chicory roots and dandelion roots are also available as powdered food supplements, which will rehydrate once in the digestive tube.

✎ Jerusalem Artichoke

Jerusalem artichoke, also known as sunchoke, is a plant in the sunflower family. At its roots it produces irregularly shaped tubers that bear a resemblance to ginger. The tubers of the Jerusalem artichoke have a slightly sweet taste that is comparable to that of artichokes, from which its most common name is derived.

Instructions for use: Jerusalem artichoke can be eaten raw, grated into a salad, or cooked.

Chicory and Dandelion Root Supplements

Manufacturer	Product
Bio Atlantic	Bio-Pissenlit (bulk dried dandelion root)
Vegavero	Dandelion Root Extract (capsules)
Penn Herb Company	Chicory Root (capsules)
MauiHerbs	Dandelion (capsules)
MauiHerbs	Chicory (capsules)
Secrets of the Tribe	Chicory (capsules)
PureNaturals	Dandelion Root (capsules)
Nutricost	Dandelion Root (capsules)
Nature's Way	Dandelion Root (capsules)

This is not an exhaustive list. (The author has no connection with, and cannot vouch for, any of the brands listed.)

Cereal Grains

Because of the many different kinds of fiber in grains and their husks, cereal grains are a good source of prebiotics.

This is true only for whole grain products, because the refining of cereal grains strips away the surface layers of the grain, which contain the bulk of the fibers.

Instructions for Use

Cereal grains can be consumed in a variety of ways—cooked whole as brown rice or barley, flakes with milk at breakfast, ground into flour for use in breads and pasta, and so on.

The grains should be whole (unrefined) and preferably organic.

PRACTICAL APPLICATION
....
Gluten Intolerance

The gluten in wheat, barley, and rye is difficult for some people to tolerate. They must refrain from using these kinds of cereal grains and eat other providers of prebiotics, such as corn, rice, millet, sorghum, quinoa, and so on, as well as potatoes and chestnuts.

Legumes

Leguminous plants (which include such foods as lentils, red beans, and so on) are also a source of prebiotics because of their high fiber content. This high content does have one drawback, however: Beans and other members of the legume family are notorious for being difficult to digest, because of their high protein, lipid, and carbohydrate content. They are therefore only recommended to people who can fully digest them.

Instructions for Use

Beans should always be eaten cooked. They combine well with cooked vegetables.

PREBIOTIC REQUIREMENTS

The recommended amount of daily prebiotic can vary greatly from one individual to another. Because the science of prebiotics is still only in its infancy, it is a good idea to simply eat generous portions of foods with prebiotic properties at every meal, and to vary the kinds of prebiotic foods you eat every day.

Nevertheless, the little test below should help you determine if your current intake of prebiotics is high enough.

Self-Diagnosis: Am I Eating Enough Fiber?

I have either whole grain bread or whole grain cereal at breakfast.	☐ Yes	☐ No
The bread I eat is whole grain bread.	☐ Yes	☐ No
I eat two to three pieces of fruit every day.	☐ Yes	☐ No
I regularly eat dried fruits.	☐ Yes	☐ No
My noon and evening meals are always accompanied by a green salad or raw vegetables.	☐ Yes	☐ No
Cooked vegetables are a regular part of my noon and evening meals.	☐ Yes	☐ No
I eat homemade soups.	☐ Yes	☐ No

Self-Diagnosis (cont.): Am I Eating Enough Fiber?

I eat brown rice.   ☐ Yes   ☐ No

I eat whole grain pasta.   ☐ Yes   ☐ No

Potatoes are a regular part of my meals.   ☐ Yes   ☐ No

I am able to digest beans easily and eat them from time to time.   ☐ Yes   ☐ No

I eat chestnuts from time to time.   ☐ Yes   ☐ No

Analysis of Results

How many *yes* answers did you have?

8 or more: Fortunately for your intestinal flora, you are eating a lot of foods that have prebiotic properties. Keep up the good work!

4–7: Your intake of prebiotics is average and your intestinal flora would be in better condition if you ate more foods with high fiber content.

3 or fewer: It is urgent that you change the way you eat so you can restore the balance of your intestinal flora.

> ### PRACTICAL APPLICATION
> ....
> #### Progress Slowly!
>
> Foods that have a high soluble fiber content gener-
> ally also contain insoluble fibers. The sensitivity of the
> intestines to these fibers varies from one person to the
> next. Someone who has rarely eaten fruits, vegetables,
> and whole grain foods and suddenly starts eating a lot
> of them may not be able to tolerate them well. They
> may experience abdominal pain, cramps, bloating, and
> diarrhea. In this case it is a good idea to reintroduce
> high-fiber foods gradually. Every individual has to move
> at whatever pace is dictated by the intestines.
>
> If there is pain, reduce the intake of high-fiber foods
> for several days. After this, gradually resume increasing
> the amount of fiber, but very cautiously. Over time the
> intestines will become accustomed to these foods that
> are high in fiber and individuals who had been sensitive
> initially can begin eating them regularly.

TWO VALUABLE SOURCES OF PREBIOTICS

Whey

Because of the lactose it contains, which is a choice food for
bacteria, whey is a prebiotic. Whey is a byproduct that comes
from making cheese. During this process the milk is curdled,
pressed, and strained. It coagulates and a hard substance

appears, which is the casein used to make cheese. The liquid produced by this procedure is whey, also called "lactoserum." It is slightly transparent and yellowish-green in color, with a slightly acidic flavor.

Using different procedures, whey can be dried into a powder or shaped into flakes. (Whey in both these forms can be found in natural food stores.) Its composition is characterized by high lactose content. In fact, while the lactose content of whole milk is less than two ounces per quart, it accounts for three-quarters of the content in whey powder.

This is why the lactose provided by whey is a choice food for the bacteria of fermentation. It has long been used to restore a healthy balance to the intestinal flora.

Instructions for Use

The whey cure is simple and makes a pleasant beverage on its own or added to a smoothie.

Mix one to two tablespoons of whey powder with one cup of water and drink three to six glasses of this mixture a day. The mixture should be consumed right away to avoid the whey turning bad. (Readers interested in learning more about the benefits of whey can read my book *The Whey Prescription,* Rochester, Vt.: Healing Arts Press, 2006.)

⚠ **Take Note!**

Whey in excess acts as a laxative. This is especially true for those who are lactose intolerant.

Lactose

Whey contains a number of nutrients: lactose, proteins, minerals, and so forth. It's possible to extract the lactose, also called "milk sugar," which converts to glucose and galactose once it has been digested and can increase the activity of intestinal microbiota.

Instructions for Use

When blended with a little water, lactose powder makes a beverage that has a pleasant and slightly sweet flavor. It can be mixed with yogurt or in desserts. It can also be used as a cure.

To use this as a remedy, mix one tablespoon of lactose powder with one cup of water three times a day. It can also be mixed with bifidus yogurt and eaten three times a day.

PRACTICAL APPLICATION
....
Dealing with Side Effects

When starting this therapy the individual may experience gas or bloating. If this is the case, take a break of one to two days, then begin again with a smaller dose (one half tablespoon) of milk sugar. You can increase this amount gradually as the corrective progresses.

PREBIOTIC SUPPLEMENTS

A number of prebiotic supplements are available commercially. The fibers they contain are no different from the fiber contained in foods. In theory these supplements are unnecessary, as simply eating enough prebiotic foods should supply the bacteria of fermentation with all the food they need. However, in practice they have been proven to be quite helpful. This is particularly true for those with sensitive intestines that become easily irritated by high fiber content, which then becomes an obstacle to eating as much fiber as they need. Taking prebiotics as a powder or in capsules can make up for this deficit.

Prebiotic Supplements

Manufacturer	Product
Bio Nutrition	Pre-Biotic
Erbology	Organic Sunchoke Powder
Lineavi	Inulin Powder
Natural Evolution	Green Banana Resistant Starch
Zestlife	Inulin
Vitamin Bounty	Prebiotic Digestive Support
BioSchwartz	Advanced Prebiotic
Hyperbiotics	Prebiotic
Gundry MD	PrebioThrive
Prebiotin	Prebiotic

Manufacturer	Product
The Granola Bakery	Inulin Powder
Microingredients	Organic Inulin Powder
Microingredients	Organic Chicory Root Inulin Powder
Ora	Trust Your Gut Vegan Probiotic & Prebiotic Supplement

This is not an exhaustive list. (The author has no connection with, and cannot vouch for, any of the brands listed.)

☕ What We've Learned

To support the intestinal flora or rebuild it from a weakened state, it is essential to provide it with the fibers, or prebiotics, that it needs to feed itself and survive. These fibers can be found in fruits, vegetables, whole grains, and beans, as well as in whey and milk sugar.

7

Repopulating the Bacteria of Fermentation with Probiotics

The regular ingestion of prebiotic fibers makes it possible to maintain a large and healthy population of flora of fermentation, and to correct any minimal, inevitable reductions in the size of its population. On the other hand, if the flora of fermentation population has been severely weakened, these maintenance procedures will not suffice. More drastic measures are required to make up for the deficit. At this critical point the intestinal flora has been decimated and it is necessary to rapidly increase the number of bacteria in residence.

In these circumstances, reconstruction of the intestinal flora is achieved by importing fermentation bacteria from outside the body to add numbers to the ones already present in the intestines. There is no waiting for bacteria to multiply, because their population is enlarged by the addition of bacteria from outside the body.

These bacteria can be consumed in two different forms. Each has its benefits and using them together is beneficial.

- Foods that have high probiotic content, such as yogurt, kefir, fresh and fermented cheeses, sauerkraut, fermented vegetables, and miso
- Probiotic supplements manufactured in a laboratory

PRACTICAL APPLICATION

What Are Probiotics?

The bacteria of fermentation are beneficial for the living, hence the name given to them of "probiotics" (literally, for life). The term can also be used to describe sources of probiotics. This is how people can speak of probiotic foods and probiotic dietary supplements. In addition, the word is used more and more to designate the probiotic food supplements that contain them. When someone talks about taking probiotics, it means taking a probiotic supplement.

PROBIOTIC FOODS

The common characteristic of probiotic foods is that they have been obtained through lactic fermentation. Lactic fermentation is a common procedure for facilitating the preservation of foods. For example, milk is preserved in the form of yogurt and cabbage is preserved in the form of sauerkraut.

Lactic fermentation is a process during which the lactic bacteria multiply by feeding on the carbohydrates provided by food. These are the same bacteria that are the predominant microorganism of the intestinal flora. They require an acidic environment in order to thrive (like the flora of fermentation in the intestines). Furthermore, their activity produces lactic acid, which helps acidify the environment in which these bacteria are present. This acidification is necessary for their survival and ability to multiply.

? Did You Know?

Lactic bacteria come from two major sources:

- External agents are added to the food intended to be preserved. This is the case with lactic starters that are mixed with milk to make yogurt, cheese, kefir, and other dairy products.

- They can originate in the food. This is the case for various kinds of vegetables that are preserved through lactic fermentation. There are not too many lactic bacteria in these foods, but they multiply liberally when the food is fermented inside a sealed container. One example is to make sauerkraut by placing cabbage inside a jar covered by a lid.

This acidity is, however, harmful to the bacteria of putrefaction that need an alkaline environment to flourish. These bacteria are hindered or even destroyed by the acidity that develops from the activity of the bacteria of fermentation. The fortunate consequence of this is that the food is no longer able to rot and decompose, so it is preserved. Food preserved this way by lactic fermentation also contains the lactic bacteria that have grown in it, and it can be a great help to our own intestinal flora when we eat food that has been preserved this way.

Regular consumption of probiotic foods is highly recommended for maintaining and supporting the beneficial flora that lives inside the intestines. It is certainly not strong enough on its own to correct severe imbalance, but it can help other efforts to restore a healthy and balanced intestinal flora.

PRACTICAL APPLICATION

For People Who Are Sensitive to Weak Acids

The majority of foods that have been preserved by lactic fermentation have a high lactic acid content. They can be recognized by their acidic taste, as is the case with sauerkraut, yogurt, pickles, and other fermented vegetables. Lactic acid is a weak acid. In bodies that are able to properly metabolize weak acids and transform them into alkaline minerals, they are a benefit. But there are people who are not able to metabolize them well. A weak acid, such as lactic acid, will consequently remain in its acidic form and cause the cellular terrain of these individuals to acidify, which can lead to numerous health disorders. (For more on this see my book *The Acid-Alkaline Diet for Optimum Health,* Rochester, Vt.: Healing Arts Press, 2006.) This is why people who have a metabolic deficiency in connection with weak acids should abstain from eating these foods, or consume them only in small quantities that are adjusted to what their bodies can tolerate.

☞ Good to Know

How can you tell if you don't metabolize weak acids well? People who are sensitive to weak acids will have sudden onsets of fatigue, red blotches on the skin, joint pain, itching, burning urination, and/or anxiety after ingesting foods rich in these acids.

Yogurt

Yogurt is probably the most well-known probiotic food. It has been a staple in the Balkans and the Middle East for many centuries. Since it became known for its health benefits and began to be manufactured by the food industry, its consumption has spread throughout the world. It is estimated to be close to fourteen pounds a year for the average American, and unfortunately that number is dropping, possibly due to an increase in easy breakfast choices. In contrast the average French citizen consumes forty-three pounds annually, followed by forty pounds a year in Switzerland and thirty-two pounds a year in Belgium.

Yogurt is obtained by causing the fermentation of lukewarm milk (108–113° F or 42–45° C), in contrast to kefir (see the section on kefir, later in this chapter), which is fermented at room temperature. The ferments that are used are two lactic bacteria: *Lactobacillus bulgaricus* and *Streptococcus thermophilus.* Additional bacteria can be added to alter the texture and flavor of the yogurt, but the Food and Drug Administration requires that both of these bacteria be present for a product to be called yogurt.

? Did You Know?

The use of probiotics for therapeutic purposes was probably started by the Russian scientist Ilya Mechnikov (1845–1916), who was awarded the Nobel Prize for medicine in 1908. His idea that bacteria could have beneficial effects on human beings was based on his observation of the health and old age attained by many elderly Bulgarians who ate yogurt daily. His research awakened great enthusiasm for Bulgarian yogurt.

The bifidus yogurts that are now most common commercially are not manufactured using these two basic kinds of bacteria. They are produced with the bacteria Bifidus regularis (a trade name) and *Lactobacillus acidophilus*. To be precise, they should not be called yogurt, but "milk that has been fermented with bifidus bacteria." In common speech, though, for the sake of convenience we still call them bifidus yogurts.

Bifidus and acidophilus bacteria are regular guests of our intestines, and the yogurts made with them have a more powerful probiotic effect than standard yogurt.

There isn't a great variety of bacteria used in making yogurt, but they are beneficial bacteria for the intestinal flora. Food regulations also stipulate that the bacteria used to manufacture yogurt must be present and alive in the final product, thereby ensuring that yogurts are active probiotics.

✪ Tips and Tricks

- To maintain intestinal flora at a healthy level, eat yogurt once or twice a day.
- If intestinal flora has been destroyed or there is treatment with antibiotics, eat three to five portions of yogurt daily.
- There can be fewer yogurt servings if the individual is consuming other probiotic products.
- Make your own yogurt at home by buying freeze-dried starter or using a starter culture.

Of course it is better if yogurt does not contain refined white sugar, and individual-serving flavored yogurts generally have high added sugar. Those who don't enjoy natural, unflavored yogurt can sweeten with honey, whole sugar, maple syrup, or fresh fruit. For those who prefer not to eat dairy or have an intolerance, soy, hemp, and coconut yogurts also provide a probiotic effect.

? Did You Know?

In addition to being a tasty addition to yogurt, honey, thanks to its FOS content, has the added benefit of a prebiotic effect.

Active Concentrates

These concentrates often have a name starting with the prefix "acti," such as Actimel made by the French company Danone, available as DanActive in the United States and Canada. They are made in much the same way as yogurt but use fermenting agents that are different from the lactobacillus variety. The final product is more concentrated than many yogurts, amounting to ten billion bacteria per serving as opposed to one billion per single-serving container of yogurt. For those seeking to maintain the current balance of their healthy intestinal flora, one serving a day is sufficient, but two to three a day is the recommended dose for a more extensive cure. These active concentrates are usually sweetened; choose the one with the lowest sugar content you can find.

Kefir

Kefir is a beverage obtained from the fermentation of milk. It is slightly fizzy, has a sour taste, and contains a very tiny amount of alcohol created by the fermentation process (less than 1 percent). It is an extremely popular beverage in Asia, Eastern Europe, and Turkey. Kefir is derived from the word *keyif* in Turkish, which means something "that gives pleasure," testifying to the fact that kefir is quite enjoyable to drink.

The fermenting agents used to manufacture kefir, called "kefir grains," look like seeds that are covered with bumps. As they grow, they start to look like small cauliflowers.

Kefir grains can contain up to thirty-four different kinds of probiotics. Ninety-five percent of these grains consist of bacteria, with yeasts making up the remaining 5 percent.

Kefir is similar to yogurt, as both are forms of fermented milk, but kefir has the consistency of a liquid. In addition, the probiotic content of kefir is much higher than that of yogurt (twenty-five to thirty billion per eight ounces).

Kefir can also be made using water and/or fruit instead of milk. The fermenting agents have different bacteria and these are less numerous, which means that water and fruit kefir are much less rich in probiotics than milk kefir.

PRACTICAL APPLICATION
....
Make Your Own Kefir

Kefir made from milk can be bought from natural food stores and some grocery stores, but it can also be made easily at home from milk and kefir grains, which are needed to start the fermentation process. Kefir grains to use with milk or ones to use with water (or coconut milk) can be purchased on the internet, at some natural food stores, and a few grocery stores. If you have your choice between dried and live, live is preferable.

- Place one tablespoon kefir grains in a quart-size glass jar.
- Pour one quart room temperature milk over the grains and cover with cheesecloth or a breathable towel, then secure with an elastic band. Note the time and let it sit at room temperature to thicken.
- Stir after twenty-four hours, use a strainer to remove the grains for use in the next batch, and refrigerate. Store the grains in water in the refrigerator.

Kefir and Lactose

Kefir contains milk but is quite low in lactose. This means that people who are lactose intolerant or particularly sensitive to it can generally tolerate the lactose in kefir. It's also possible that consumption of kefir will improve the ability to tolerate lactose.

Instructions for Use

Drink every day as a pleasant beverage or as part of a cure consisting of one liter per day for one month.

Fermented Cheeses

Fermented cheeses such as cheddar, comté, camembert, gouda, mozzarella, and blue cheese are high in probiotics.

The first stage in manufacturing these cheeses is curdling the milk with fermenting agents or rennet. Contrary to what one might think, it is not the fermenting agents that give cheese its high probiotic content. This high content is developed after the stages of draining and salting of the curds, which is most simply known as the aging process.

The aging process is a ripening process during which the bacteria contained in the curds multiply. This bacterial activity gradually transforms the curd mixture through fermentation into cheese. It changes in consistency, odor, flavor, and so forth. A crust also forms on the surface. The active bacteria in this process are *Lactobacillus thermophilus, Lactobacillus bulgaricus, Lactobacillus acidophilus,* and so on.

During the course of this ripening process that can range from several months to quite often more than a year, depending on the kind of cheese, the fermentation bacteria multiply. This is how, as it ages and ripens, the bacteria population in the cheese increases, which enhances its probiotic properties.

Depending on the manufacturing processes employed, three different kinds of cheese can be obtained.

- *Soft Cheeses:* The drained and salted curds are immediately placed in a mold and left to ferment. The cheese becomes soft and a rind forms on the outside. The crust develops a white fuzzy surface, thanks to the activity of molds. Cheeses in this category include camembert, brie, Muenster, Pont-L'Évêque, and others. The last two cheeses mentioned do not have a white rind because the mold is brushed off the surface during the aging process.
- *Hard Cheeses:* The drained and salted cheese is placed in a mold, but unlike the manufacturing process used for soft cheeses, the curd mixture is pressed. This ensures that these cheeses are harder than the previous category because they contain less water. Some of the cheeses found in the hard cheese category are comté, gruyère, parmesan, gouda, edam, and cheddar.
- *Blue-Veined Cheeses:* The drained and salted curds are placed in a mold but not pressed. To the contrary, strains of yeast are injected into the mass by long needles to obtain a fermentation process that starts from the inside. The cheese produced by this method is crumbly and has a strong, peppery taste. Scattered throughout it are clumps and veins of blue or green colored yeast. Some of the cheeses in this category are blue cheese, Roquefort, Gorgonzola, and Stilton.

Instructions for Use

The cheeses mentioned above are concentrated foods and highly nutritious. It would be a mistake to try to eat large amounts of these cheeses in order to obtain more probiotics, as it would cause digestive problems. However, there is no reason that cheese cannot be a part of your regular diet. For example, you might enjoy cheese two or three times a week as a way to help maintain the intestinal flora, or daily as part of a more intense corrective when the intestinal flora is greatly unbalanced.

Fresh Cheeses

The production of fresh cheeses is much simpler. For these cheeses the milk is fermented with the help of various lactic fermenting agents. The curd that results is more or less drained, then eaten as is without salting or aging. The multiplication of lactic bacteria that happens during the ripening of aged cheeses does not occur. The probiotic content of fresh cheeses is entirely due to the multiplication of these bacteria during the curdling process. It is consequently much lower than that of fermented cheeses.

Cheeses in this category include feta, fromage blanc, cottage cheese, ricotta, mascarpone, quark, cream cheese, and so on.

Instructions for Use

Fresh cheeses have 80 percent water content as opposed to the 30 percent average of hard cheeses. They are therefore much less concentrated foods and can be eaten daily and in larger quantities.

Sauerkraut

Sauerkraut is made by sprinkling thinly sliced cabbage leaves with salt and placing them in a sealed container. The bacteria that are naturally present in the cabbage leaves produce a lactic acid that give the final product its sour flavor.

The active bacteria are primarily *Lactobacillus plantarum* and *Lactobacillus cucumeris* as well as *Leuconostoc mesenteroides*. In addition to its very high content of lactic bacteria, sauerkraut contains a large number of enzymes. Both of these characteristics explain why sauerkraut possesses such propitious properties for digestion. This is most likely why it is often eaten with fatty meats and sausages, but is also regularly used—as a side dish—by people who have poor digestion.

The beneficial activity of sauerkraut for the intestinal flora is twofold:

- It imports a large number of probiotic bacteria into the intestines, thereby allowing the intestinal flora to regenerate.
- It brings in lactic acid that makes the intestinal environment more acidic, preventing the survival and proliferation of the putrefaction bacteria.

? Did You Know?

Enzymes are *not* probiotics. Both transform matter, but probiotics are single-celled living organisms whereas enzymes are only protein substances with specific properties.

✛ Tips and Tricks

There are more probiotics in sauerkraut that is raw.

Instructions for Use

It is better to eat sauerkraut frequently in small quantities as an accompaniment to other dishes, rather than eating large amounts of it from time to time. It can be eaten by itself or with raw vegetables, or even included in a green or mixed salad.

Lactic Fermentation of Vegetables

The same procedure used for making sauerkraut can be used for preserving other vegetables. Some of the primary vegetables prepared this way include pickles, pearl onions, olives, beets, carrots, garlic, and lemons.

✛ Tips and Tricks

To benefit from the probiotic effect of fermented foods, make certain they were really prepared by a lactic fermentation process and not simply pickled in vinegar to give them a sour flavor.

Instructions for Use

These kinds of foods can be eaten whenever your menu includes compatible dishes. They do not provide a large number of probiotics but are nonetheless beneficial for maintaining the balance of the intestinal flora.

Juices Made
by Lactic Fermentation

Some of the juices sold commercially have been preserved by means of lactic fermentation (as is always stated on the label). These juices consequently have a sour and very pleasant taste.

Instructions for Use

Can be enjoyed whenever you wish to have a refreshing beverage.

Miso

Miso is a traditional food of Japan that has become increasingly popular in Europe and North America over the past several decades. It is a thick paste with a texture quite similar to peanut butter. Depending on what variety it is, miso can be white to red to deep brown in color. It has a pleasant flavor but is also strong and rather salty.

Miso is made from soybeans and rice or barley, as well as water and salt. Lactic fermentation agents and special fungi— *Aspergillus oryzae, Aspergillus sojae*—are added to this blend of ingredients.

Instructions for Use

There are many different ways that miso can be used:

- Miso soup
- As a seasoning
- In sauces and salad dressing
- As a spread or dip

Kombucha

The slightly fizzy, sour-flavored beverage known as kombucha has become increasingly popular. It is prepared by fermenting black tea, green tea, or herbal tea with the addition of a combination of sugar and a special blend of bacteria and yeast called a SCOBY (symbiotic colony of bacteria and yeast). This blend is sold commercially and makes it possible to make kombucha at home, something that can be done repeatedly for years as the SCOBY can be reused.

Natural food stores and organic supermarkets sell bottled kombucha beverages.

? Did You Know?

There are many health benefits attributed to kombucha. In Chinese, its name means "elixir of immortality." Its high content of probiotics certainly contributes to its good reputation.

Instructions for Use

Kombucha is a pleasant beverage that can be consumed at any time.

Other Sources of Probiotics

There are other foods that are sources of probiotics because the process used to make them involves fermentation:

- Soy sauce
- Sourdough bread
- Brottrunk, a beverage made from fermented bread must
- Kvass, a beverage made from fermented rye or black bread
- Tempeh, made from fermented soybeans
- Kimchi, a Korean version of sauerkraut made with cabbage and other vegetables
- Natto, made from fermented soybeans

PROBIOTIC SUPPLEMENTS

Probiotic supplements are a great help when the intestinal flora has been severely damaged and its population decimated, for example by antibiotics. Probiotic supplements can supply as many as 550 billion bacteria per gel cap. This supply is therefore of a completely different order from that offered by foods with probiotic properties. Yogurt, for example, generally contains a maximum of one billion bacteria per serving. Probiotic supplements are therapy, whereas probiotic foods are still in the dietary domain. However, foods are much more effective over the long term.

The bacteria contained in probiotic supplements are primarily lactic bacteria of the *Bifidobacterium* and *Lactobacillus* genera. These strains are strongly represented in the flora of fermentation, but other kinds of bacteria are also used.

The Official Definition of Probiotics

The World Health Organization has defined probiotics as "live microorganisms, which, when administered in adequate amounts, confer a health benefit on the host."

The living bacteria used to make health supplements must be prepared with this purpose in mind. They are gently freeze-dried and placed in a state of suspended animation, as if they were "put to sleep." They are still alive but no longer exhibit any activity, which makes it possible to preserve them. The water-removal process used to achieve this result is called "lyophilization." Bacteria selected for this process are first frozen at a temperature of –22°F, then dried at between 59° and 86°F. When these supplements are ingested, these bacteria enter the moist, warm environment of the intestines and awaken from their torpor. They then recover full vitality and become active again.

Criteria for Probiotics

In order to be useful, bacteria contained in probiotic supplements have to arrive alive in the lower half of the small intestine and in the ascending colon, the places where they will be put to use. In order to ensure this, the bacteria selected must be manufactured according to a certain number of criteria.

1. The bacteria must be *living* so that once they arrive in the intestines they are able to become active.
2. The bacteria must not only still be alive upon ingestion, they must be still living when they reach the intestines and colon. What this means is that they must be capable of resisting the gastric acidity that could otherwise kill them.
3. The bacteria must reach their destination in the intestines in sufficient numbers that when they multiply they outweigh the excessive bacteria of putrefaction or any pathological bacteria that may be present (barrier effect).
4. The bacteria selected must be natural residents of the intestines so they are capable of surviving in this environment. Having the ability to adapt to the living conditions that govern this region, they will be able to multiply and work in a way that is beneficial.
5. The bacteria must be able to attach themselves to the intestinal walls (at least temporarily) for two reasons: so they are not transported out of this area by the stools and possibly eliminated from the body, which would reduce their numbers, making the work of the remaining bacteria less effective; and because when they occupy an area they prevent harmful bacteria from taking that space.

Depending on the bacteria that have been selected and the care given to the manufacture of the supplements, probiotic complexes will be active to a greater or lesser degree, which will determine how effective they are.

PRACTICAL APPLICATION

Who Should Take a Probiotic Cure?

People who most need a probiotic cure are those who suffer from

- Recurring digestive problems: diarrhea, indigestion, irritable bowel syndrome, constipation, and so forth
- Repeated infections: fungal infections, cystitis, colds, and so on
- Allergies
- Side effects of antibiotics
- Psychological problems: anxiety, depression, and so forth

How Effective Are Probiotics?

In the best-case scenarios, bacteria in probiotic supplements will make their way to the bottom half of the small intestine and the ascending colon, and once there manage to attach themselves to the intestinal walls. This act of attaching themselves to the walls of the intestines is crucial; it provides them support and allows them to expand. Even if some of these bacteria are carried out of the body with the stool, a certain number that have anchored themselves solidly to the walls will remain. Here they will begin to multiply and provide a replacement population for the deficient bacteria of fermentation, which is the basic cause of the imbalance of the intestinal flora. They are now a part of this flora and their activity will have long-term results.

Most often, however, this best-case scenario is not the case: the probiotic bacteria are not able to affix themselves to the intestinal walls or multiply. Yet having successfully reached their destination they will be put to work and survive in their new environment. They won't manage to get established but their presence creates a barrier effect that slows the bacteria of putrefaction. This will allow the bacteria of fermentation that are already established in the intestines to rebuild and multiply.

Benefits of Probiotics

Although bacteria from probiotics do not remain permanently in the intestines, their temporary presence offers a number of benefits:

- They increase the population of the flora of fermentation, thus slowing proliferation of the bacteria of putrefaction or pathogenic bacteria (the barrier effect).
- Any probiotic bacteria that do manage to attach themselves to the intestinal walls, even if only temporarily, prevent pathogenic bacteria from establishing themselves there.
- They neutralize the aggressive toxins that are released by harmful bacteria. This protects not only the intestines but the rest of the body against allergies, inflammation, and other health disorders.

- Because they are bacteria of fermentation, they produce acids that create the slightly acidic pH necessary for the healthy development of beneficial intestinal flora, but block the establishment of the bacteria of putrefaction.
- Some bacteria have "foreign" characteristics. They consequently compel the microbiota to remain vigilant and ready to take quick action, which strengthens it and makes it more efficient.
- The presence of these alien bacteria stimulates the mucous membranes to produce protective mucus in higher quantities and better quality. Moreover, this protective activity also works against pathogenic bacteria in general. This increases the body's opportunities to defend itself.

Several Important Observations

There are several important points that can be taken from what we have just discussed here:

1. Taking probiotics is less about rebuilding the flora of fermentation than it is about giving the existing flora an opportunity to rebuild itself.
2. A probiotic cure is only effective when the flora of fermentation have been weakened or destroyed.
3. When the intestinal flora is balanced, probiotic supplements have no effect and are therefore useless.
4. The effect of probiotic supplements lasts only as long as the cure.

✛ Tips and Tricks

Probiotic supplements, even those extremely high in bacteria that promise long-lasting action, are not effective in regenerating the intestinal flora unless the diet changes at the same time to one with high prebiotic fiber content.

Different Forms of Probiotics

Because all the bacteria used for manufacturing probiotic supplements have been freeze-dried, they are in the form of a dry powder. It is only when these bacteria are in the warm and moist environment of our intestines that they become active again.

Probiotic supplements are available in several different forms.

Powders

Bacteria that have been freeze-dried (lyophilized) into a powder form is usually packaged in small packets that correspond to a single dose. Sometimes the powder is sold loose in a larger package and the dose is determined by a measuring spoon or a simple household spoon.

The powder is mixed in cold or lukewarm water, then drunk. Because it is a liquid support medium, the bacteria don't remain for long in the stomach but rapidly make their way into the intestines. The stomach actually has the propensity, in accordance with its role, to retain all solids for digestion and expel all liquids into the intestines. As this is the case, it is a good idea to take a probiotic preparation before meals, when the stomach is empty. There is one additional advantage to taking this supplement before eating: because the stomach has not yet released any digestive juices, the quantity of acid that has the potential to kill the probiotic bacteria is smaller.

Soft Capsules

In this form, the probiotic bacteria have been packaged in soft gelatin capsules. They dissolve very easily in the intestines.

As a general rule, one capsule is equal to one dose, but sometimes it may be necessary to take several capsules at one time.

Gelcaps

Gelcaps are harder than gelatin capsules. They have an outer covering that consists of several layers and therefore they take much longer to dissolve. This helps ensure that the bacteria are not released until they have reached the lower regions of the intestines. The bacteria have a better chance of survival because they do not come into direct contact with the acidity of the stomach.

How to Choose a Probiotic Supplement

There are many probiotic supplements available. Which is the best one for you among this abundance of products? Which will be the most effective for you?

A great help for determining the answer to these questions is knowing the characteristic differences among the different kinds. Here are a few criteria on which to base your decision.

Probiotic supplements distinguish themselves from each other by:

The Number of Probiotic Bacteria

The higher the number of bacteria present in the supplement, the higher the number likely to survive the journey to the lower intestines and the more beneficial the supplement will be. The bacteria are measured in CFUs (colony forming units). A CFU can vary from five to one hundred billion bacteria. These figures make it possible to make helpful comparisons of the various products.

When you consider that the average bacteria content of a serving of yogurt is one billion CFUs and kefir has twenty-five to thirty billion CFUs, you might ask yourself if it is worth the trouble to take a probiotic supplement with a dosage of five billion CFUs. The answer is yes, provided that the coating protects the bacteria and increases the likelihood they will still be alive when they reach the intestines.

Types of Bacteria

There are many different types of beneficial bacteria. The bacteria most often present in supplements are lactobacillus and bifidobacteria, separate or together. Depending on the product, they may be combined with other bacteria. But there are also preparations that consist of only other bacteria.

? Did You Know?

Lactose intolerance is not a contraindication. The bacteria most often used in probiotic supplements is *Lactobacillus,* and although it's found in milk, it's not milk and does not contain lactose.

The bacteria in different probiotic supplements are always listed by name on the label. For example, you might see *"Lactobacillus rhamnosus* GG." How are we supposed to interpret this name or one like it?

The first name that appears, *Lactobacillus,* indicates the genus of the bacteria. The second part of the name, *rhamnosus,* designates the species within the *Lactobacillus* genus. There can be hundreds, or more precisely thousands, of different species within one genus of bacteria. The third indicator is either a number or letters, in this case GG. These indicate the strain of bacteria within the species.

Using this as our guide, we can see that *Lactobacillus rhamnosus* and *Lactobacillus helveticus* are from the same genus but belong to different species. On the other hand, *Lactobacillus rhamnosus* GG R00343 and *Lactobacillus rhamnosus* R0011 are similar when it comes to genus and species but are not from the same strain.

A precise designation is important because each type of bacteria, based on its species or strain, possesses unique properties. Unfortunately, the FDA does not require labels to include strain designations or viable counts on yogurt or probiotics. However, efforts are now being made to improve labeling and facilitate transparency.

The Targeted Health Problem

All probiotic supplements share the same goal of rebuilding the intestinal flora of fermentation. In the past, reconstruction of this flora was the sole objective for taking supplements. A better understanding of the properties of the different strains has now expanded the range of activity for these preparations.

Depending on their composition, they can have as an additional complementary therapeutic action for the following:

- Diarrhea
- Digestive weakness
- Constipation
- Irritable bowel
- Fungal infections
- Travel abroad
- Immune system weakness
- Weight loss

Variety of Strains

While the total number of bacteria is important, the number of different strains—their variety—is equally significant. Because each strain of bacteria has different functions, different supplements have a different spectrum of activity.

The Addition of Prebiotics or Not

Because bacteria feed on prebiotics, some manufacturers have combined fibers in the form of inulin, FOS, or GOS with the freeze-dried bacteria, so that these bacteria, as soon as they come back to life inside the intestines, have nutrients at their immediate disposal. This addition should not be a deciding factor, as there should be generous quantities of fiber in the intestines of everyone who regularly eats fruits and vegetables. Probiotics with prebiotics included are specifically recommended for people who do not include much fiber in their diet.

Gelcap Coating

Gelcaps and soft capsules traditionally have been made from bovine or porcine gelatin. There are now capsules made from plant-based material, some gluten-free, starch-free, sugar-free, and so on.

How Do I Take Probiotics?

General instructions are offered here for how to proceed with probiotics. For specific instructions please follow the information provided by the product's manufacturer.

When Do I Take Them?

As a general rule probiotics are taken before meals when the stomach is empty, so that they can make their way into the intestines more quickly. But the transit of probiotic supplements through the stomach can be uncomfortable for some people. In this case it's a better idea to take them during the meal to prevent them from making contact with the stomach lining.

Expiration Date

All probiotic supplements have an expiration date. Make sure you buy and use them before their sell-by date. The bacteria may have been freeze-dried into a state of suspended animation, but that does not mean they won't change over time.

Storage

Respect the manufacturer's instructions concerning the storage of probiotic supplements. Some can be stored at room temperature but others will have to be refrigerated. In no case should they be exposed to sunlight or any source of heat.

Dosage

Dosage varies from one supplement to the next. Please follow the instructions recommended by the manufacturer.

Length of the Cure

Intensive cures will last from one week to several months. Following a course of treatment, it is a good idea to solidify the results by continuing to take one to two doses a week for a period of two to three months. The same amount is also recommended for a preventative dose. If you find after a month that the corrective is not doing its job, it could be that the bacteria in the preparation you are taking are not the bacteria you need. In this case you should switch to another probiotic supplement.

Side Effects

There are no side effects from taking probiotics. At the very most some extra-sensitive individuals might start feeling one of the following symptoms: minor stomach discomfort, gas, bloating, or constipation. This is usually remedied by taking the supplement during meals, rather than before them.

How Long Does It Take for Beneficial Effects to Begin?

The speed with which the effects start to appear depends on the degree of the initial health problem. While the effects countering some conditions—for example, infectious diarrhea (gastroenteritis)—begin to show up in just a few hours, it usually takes at least a week to feel any improvement from well-established disorders. But these will be only the first signs of improvement. A full cure usually takes several weeks or even a month, depending on the individual case.

Several Examples of Probiotics

For the sole purpose of facilitating the reader's first steps into the world of probiotics, I am providing a list here of companies that produce good-quality probiotic supplements. However, this list is far from being exhaustive. There are many, many other supplements available. I would also like to stress that I have no connection with any of the brands listed.

The first column lists the names of the companies in alphabetical order. The second column lists the name of one of the supplements they produce. Many companies manufacture several different kinds of probiotics.

Company	Product
Be-Life	Bifibiol
Bio-Life	Advanced Multiblend Probiotix
Burgerstein	Biotics-G
Carrare	Bioprotus
A. Vogel	Aciforce Probioticum
Fenioux	Optiflorus
Le Stum	Lactospectrum
MegaFood	MegaFlora
Nutergia	Ergyphilus Plus
Pharmalp	Pharmalp Pro-P
PharmaNutrics	Proflore Plus
PiLeJe	Lactibiane
Yves Ponroy	Entéroflore
Renew Life	Ultimate Flora
Sanofi	Bioflorin
Töpfer	Eugalan Forte
Vit'All+	Acidophilus+Biofidus
Vita Miracle	Ultra-30 Probiotics
Xantis	Flore
Yalacta	Sécuril

🎓 What We've Learned

To encourage reconstruction of the intestinal flora, individuals may ingest bacteria of fermentation—in the form of probiotics—that will join the existing flora. This can be done by consuming:

- Foods with high probiotic content
- Probiotic supplements, which contain billions of bacteria that have been lyophilized (freeze-dried)

8

Reducing the Flora of Putrefaction

The fermentation flora and the putrefaction flora have a symbiotic relationship. What happens to one will have immediate repercussions upon the other, so when the numbers of flora of fermentation are reduced an automatic increase in the flora of putrefaction follows. Not only will the size of this latter flora grow larger but it will also expand into areas of the colon where it should not be present: the right half of the transverse colon and the ascending colon, regions normally reserved for the bacteria of fermentation. Once there, the putrefaction bacteria will also alter the pH of these regions and make it slightly alkaline, which is self-serving but hinders development of the flora of fermentation.

A diet rich in prebiotics along with the ingestion of probiotics rebuilds the flora of fermentation over the long haul and gives it the means it needs to reconquer those parts of the colon that are naturally reserved for it. But sometimes this process is too slow and needs some help to reduce the flora of putrefaction more quickly. There are ways to do this.

CHANGE YOUR DIET

An imbalance of the intestinal flora that benefits the flora of putrefaction is only possible when the bacteria of putrefaction have enough food to develop and multiply. Deprived of the food they depend on, they weaken and die, and their reduced numbers start to correspond to what should be the normal population of the flora of putrefaction. Foods that increase growth of the bacteria of putrefaction are high in protein, such as meat and fish, but also cheese and eggs. The typical diet includes large amounts of protein at every meal, which is extremely favorable for the bacteria of putrefaction. It is this kind of diet that needs to be changed.

The change to a better diet consists of drastically reducing—at least 50 percent if not more—consumption of meat and fish. A reduction of the quantity of cheese and eggs is also necessary. Ultimately this means adopting a diet that is 80 percent plant-based foods and no more than 20 percent animal-based foods.

PRACTICAL APPLICATION
....
**Reduce Sugar to
Reduce Putrefaction Flora**

White sugar, sweets (candies, chocolate, pastry, ice cream, and so on), and fats (fried foods and butter) are as destructive in the microbiota as an excess of proteins, if not more so. The consumption of these foods also has to be greatly reduced—if not eliminated outright—to reduce the size of the flora of putrefaction and encourage regeneration of the flora of fermentation.

ENEMAS

The concentration of the bacteria of putrefaction is always greatest in the descending colon. This is why enemas are a good way to get rid of excessive numbers of these bacteria. The water that is introduced into the colon will liquefy its contents so that the stools are expelled much more easily, carrying with them the putrefaction flora located there. Simply by using enemas several times, you will greatly reduce the population of the flora of putrefaction.

Isn't there a risk of destroying too much of these bacteria? No, there is already too much and enemas will simply reduce their numbers, not eliminate them completely. Furthermore, those that have affixed themselves to the colon walls will renew this flora when they begin multiplying.

☝ Good to Know

Enemas are only active on the descending colon. They don't disturb the fermentation flora, which is higher up in the intestines. This is not the case for purges, which completely empty the intestines—small and large.

The reduction of the flora of putrefaction will weaken the barrier effect it has on the flora of fermentation, making it easier for the flora of fermentation to win back its rightful territory in the colon (that is, the ascending colon and first half of the transverse colon).

Where to Get an Enema

An enema can be administered by a colon hydrotherapist in a comfortable, professional setting or self-administered in the privacy of your home.

Home Enema

The quantity of liquid needed to do an enema is two liters—a little more than two quarts. This volume of water will fill the rectum and the descending colon.

The equipment required for a home enema can be found in drugstores and pharmacies. An enema kit will include a measuring container for the water, a long rubber tube, and a cannula with a valve.

✚ Tips and Tricks

The water temperature for an enema should be in the neighborhood of 98.6°F. If the water is too cold it will cause abdominal cramps; if it is too warm it will be unpleasantly hot or even scald the colon. Tap water is perfectly suitable.

Application

The container filled with water should be placed higher than the individual, on a table or shelf, so the water can easily enter the intestines. The cannula with its valve closed is inserted into the anus. Once the individual is on all fours with head and torso leaning forward, the valve of the cannula can be opened.

After the water has been introduced into the colon, the cannula is removed. The liquid must be retained in the colon for a fairly good time (five to ten minutes) in order for the stools to become thoroughly liquefied. The individual can facilitate the irrigation of the colon either by inhaling deeply from the diaphragm or by slightly shifting position.

After this interval the individual should sit on a toilet in order to empty the liquid that was injected and the matter that has been dissolved into it.

To achieve a more thorough and powerful effect, it is recommended to do a series of three enemas in fairly close succession. That means every two days. After this the enemas should be continued with one enema a week for three weeks.

🎓 What We've Learned

The reduction of an overgrown population of the bacteria of putrefaction can be done in two different ways:

- By depriving them of the food they need to thrive and multiply, which means reducing consumption of meat, white sugar, and fats
- By doing enemas that will carry large numbers of these bacteria out of the body

Conclusion

A strong and balanced intestinal flora does not depend on remedies or sophisticated treatments, but primarily on a healthy lifestyle. This is a parameter we can work within easily. It doesn't take high-priced supplements or expensive therapies, only simple adjustments to our daily diet.

The benefit is overall better health. There are countless recommendations for health improvement but the simple fact of balancing our microbiota through more thoughtful food intake can leave us with more energy and stamina.

The foods that balance our intestinal flora are far from the most expensive. It's up to us to make smart and healthy choices about what goes into our grocery baskets, and consequently into our bodies.

The COVID-19 pandemic is a forceful reminder of the importance of keeping our immune systems in peak condition. A balanced microbiota is no guarantee against infection and illness, but it helps our bodies to fend off any pathogens that come our way.

This happy equilibrium will be profoundly reflected in our physical and mental well-being.

Index

BOOKS OF RELATED INTEREST

Freedom from Constipation
Natural Remedies for Digestive Health
by Christopher Vasey, N.D.

Good Sugar, Bad Sugar
How to Power Your Body and Brain with Healthy Energy
by Christopher Vasey, N.D.

The Acid–Alkaline Diet for Optimum Health
Restore Your Health by Creating pH Balance in Your Diet
by Christopher Vasey, N.D.

Liver Detox
Cleansing through Diet, Herbs, and Massage
by Christopher Vasey, N.D.

Natural Remedies for Inflammation
by Christopher Vasey, N.D.

Natural Antibiotics and Antivirals
18 Infection-Fighting Herbs and Essential Oils
by Christopher Vasey, N.D.

The Water Prescription
For Health, Vitality, and Rejuvenation
by Christopher Vasey, N.D.

Cultivating Your Microbiome
Ayurvedic and Chinese Practices for a Healthy Gut
and a Clear Mind
by Bridgette Shea, L.Ac., MAcOM

INNER TRADITIONS • BEAR & COMPANY
P.O. Box 388 • Rochester, VT 05767
1-800-246-8648 • www.InnerTraditions.com

Or contact your local bookseller